Dear Reader,

When I first started my career as a dietitian, FODMAPs weren't something I had heard of yet. When the term started making its way around my professional circles, I knew it was only a matter of time before my clients started asking about it. After my first review of the low-FODMAP diet, I was overwhelmed! Not only was there a lot of information about how to follow this diet, but it also felt daunting that there seemed to be more foods to remove than there were **foods to enjoy**.

I didn't want my clients to feel this way, so I decided to learn as much as I could about this diet. What I discovered is that this approach is **highly individualized** and requires a lot of trial and error. What works for one person on their low-FODMAP journey may not be what works for another. Working with a trained nutrition professional who has expertise in FODMAPs will help you manage your gastrointestinal (GI) symptoms and set you on the path to having control over your gut.

My goal is always to help someone be as minimally restrictive with the greatest symptom resolution. Simply put, the goal of the low-FODMAP diet is not complete elimination of higher-FODMAP foods permanently. Think of it as testing your limits. Knowing which foods (and what amounts) are manageable for you **gives you all the power** you need over your symptoms.

The recipes in this cookbook are designed to make the transition to a low-FODMAP diet easy. Plus, these recipes are **delicious options** that your whole family can enjoy. Following a low-FODMAP diet doesn't have to be bland, boring, or scary, or feel like a punishment. With this book, your transition to a low-FODMAP life will be filled with flavorful meals and tasty treats.

Melinda Boyd, DCN, RD, FAND

Welcome to the Everything® Series!

These handy, accessible books give you all you need to tackle a difficult project, gain a new hobby, comprehend a fascinating topic, prepare for an exam, or even brush up on something you learned back in school but have since forgotten.

You can choose to read an Everything® book from cover to cover or just pick out the information you want from our four useful boxes: Questions, Facts, Alerts, and Essentials. We give you everything you need to know on the subject, but throw in a lot of fun stuff along the way too.

question	fact
Answers to common questions.	Important snippets of information.

alert	essential
Urgent warnings.	Quick handy tips.

We now have more than 600 Everything® books in print, spanning such wide-ranging categories as cooking, health, parenting, personal finance, wedding planning, word puzzles, and so much more. When you're done reading them all, you can finally say you know Everything®!

PUBLISHER Karen Cooper

MANAGING EDITOR Lisa Laing

ASSOCIATE COPY DIRECTOR Casey Ebert

PRODUCTION EDITOR Jo-Anne Duhamel

ACQUISITIONS EDITOR Julia Belkas

DEVELOPMENT EDITOR Brett Palana-Shanahan

EVERYTHING® SERIES COVER DESIGNER Erin Alexander

THE

EVERYTHING®

Easy

Low-FODMAP Diet
Cookbook

175 Healthy Recipes to Reduce Digestive Symptoms, Improve Gut Health, and Feel Your Best

Colleen Francioli, RN
With Melinda Boyd, DCN, RD, FAND

ADAMS MEDIA

NEW YORK   AMSTERDAM/ANTWERP   LONDON   TORONTO
SYDNEY/MELBOURNE   NEW DELHI

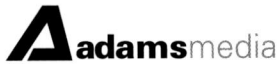

Aadamsmedia

Adams Media
An Imprint of Simon & Schuster, LLC
100 Technology Center Drive
Stoughton, MA 02072

For more than 100 years, Simon & Schuster has championed authors and the stories they create. By respecting the copyright of an author's intellectual property, you enable Simon & Schuster and the author to continue publishing exceptional books for years to come. We thank you for supporting the author's copyright by purchasing an authorized edition of this book.

An Everything® Series Book.

Everything® and everything.com® are registered trademarks of Simon & Schuster, LLC.

First Adams Media trade paperback edition January 2026

ADAMS MEDIA and colophon are registered trademarks of Simon & Schuster, LLC.

Simon & Schuster strongly believes in freedom of expression and stands against censorship in all its forms. For more information, visit BooksBelong.com.

For information about special discounts for bulk purchases, please contact Simon & Schuster Special Sales at 1-866-506-1949 or business@simonandschuster.com.

The Simon & Schuster Speakers Bureau can bring authors to your live event. For more information or to book an event, contact the Simon & Schuster Speakers Bureau at 1-866-248-3049 or visit our website at www.simonspeakers.com.

Interior design by Maya Caspi
Photographs by Emily Weeks

Manufactured in the United States of America

10 9 8 7 6 5 4 3 2 1

Library of Congress Cataloging-in-Publication Data has been applied for.

ISBN 978-1-5072-2567-7
ISBN 978-1-5072-2568-4 (ebook)

Always follow safety and commonsense cooking protocols while using kitchen utensils, operating ovens and stoves, and handling uncooked food. If children are assisting in the preparation of any recipe, they should always be supervised by an adult.

The information in this book should not be used for diagnosing or treating any health problem. Not all diet and exercise plans suit everyone. You should always consult a trained medical professional before starting a diet, taking any form of medication, or embarking on any fitness or weight training program. The author and publisher disclaim any liability arising directly or indirectly from the use of this book.

Contains material adapted from the following title published by Adams Media, an Imprint of Simon & Schuster, LLC: *The Everything® Low-FODMAP Diet Cookbook* by Colleen Francioli, CNC, copyright © 2016, ISBN 978-1-4405-9529-5.

Contents

Introduction

If you are reading this cookbook, it's likely that you or a loved one has been told to go on a low-FODMAP diet. Or perhaps bloating, gas, and digestive issues have been causing you distress and you've heard about the benefits a low-FODMAP diet can have for your gut health. Whatever your reason, you should know that you're not alone. Incidents of IBS and gut-related issues are on the rise, and that means more people than ever are looking for delicious recipes that will keep them satisfied and free from pain. Fortunately, there's no need to miss out on the foods you love due to IBS, a food allergy or intolerance, or other digestive problems. With *The Everything® Easy Low-FODMAP Diet Cookbook*, you can enjoy delicious foods that not only fulfill your cravings but keep you feeling healthy and well!

From hearty breakfasts and tantalizing dinners to desserts of all kinds, the 175 recipes in this book are diverse, delicious, and easy to prepare—and best of all, they require only simple, everyday ingredients, so you don't have to spend your valuable time running out to the store. With step-by-step instructions and handy tips and suggestions, eating on the low-FODMAP diet has never been easier!

Inside, you'll find new, healthier versions of your favorite foods that you'll want to make again and again, such as:

- Raspberry Lemon Oatmeal Bars
- Feta Cheese Dip
- Chicken Tortilla Soup
- Mediterranean Buckwheat Salad
- Roast Beef Tenderloin with Parmesan Crust
- Goat Cheese and Potato Tacos with Red Chili Cream Sauce
- Seafood Risotto
- Carrot Cake with Cream Cheese Frosting
- And so much more!

In addition, in order to avoid the common fillers and additives (which may harm your gut health) found in many store-bought foods, you'll discover how to make your own basic pantry staples from scratch, including mayonnaise, ketchup, tomato sauces, salad dressings and marinades, gluten-free breads, pizza dough, egg replacers, and more.

You'll also find important information on how to transition to eating on the low-FODMAP diet, including the elimination and challenge phases. Chapter 1 will look at what FODMAPs are, the conditions that can benefit most from this diet, and how to track your eating and symptoms. At the end of the book, you'll also find helpful meal plans and snack suggestions to make low-FODMAP eating even easier.

Whether you're new to the low-FODMAP diet or just looking for new, gut-friendly ideas, you'll find plenty of delicious recipes, along with valuable information to help you take charge of your health journey, in this book. Eating a low-FODMAP diet doesn't mean missing out on your favorite foods or fun events. This handy guide provides inspiration to cook delicious, flavorful dishes, all while bettering your body, mind, and—of course—gut.

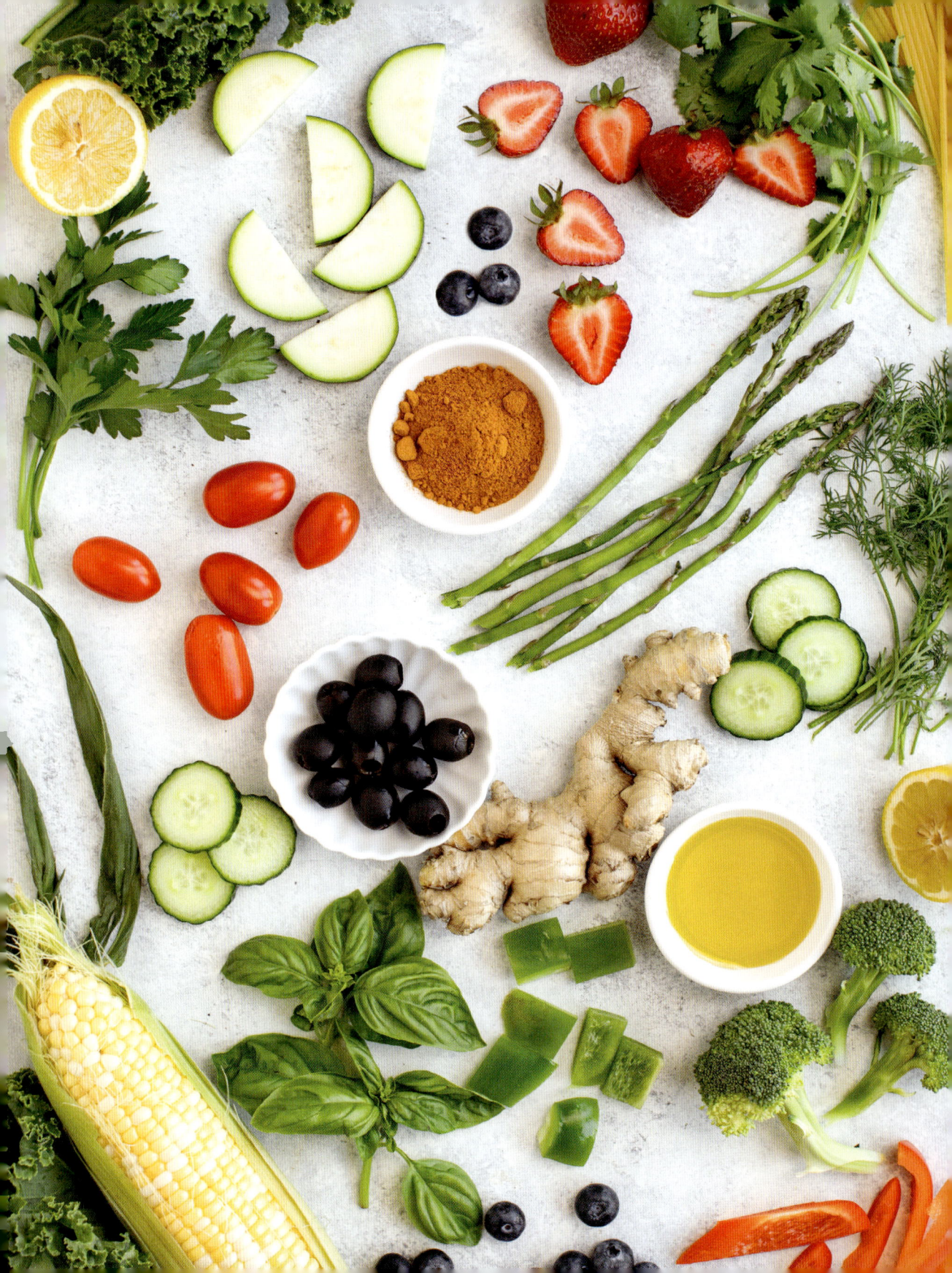

CHAPTER 1

What Is the Low-FODMAP Diet?

The low-FODMAP diet is an elimination diet designed to help people who endure symptoms of irritable bowel syndrome (IBS) and other digestive issues. This plan is a dietary approach to IBS, and it can help you identify common foods you eat regularly that may be triggering issues in your body. The diet focuses on food components known as FODMAPs (fermentable oligosaccharides, disaccharides, monosaccharides, and polyols)—components that contribute to digestive symptoms in people with IBS. Ultimately, this diet will help you identify and eliminate the types of FODMAPs that are causing your problems and get you to a place where you can enjoy a wide range of foods with the greatest symptom reduction.

The History of the Low-FODMAP Diet

In 1999, after years of witnessing her patients with celiac disease and difficult-to-treat symptoms suffer, Accredited Practicing Dietitian Dr. Sue Shepherd studied the role of fructose and fructans in gut symptoms and developed what she called the fructose malabsorption diet. Years later, after looking at the role of *other* poorly absorbed food components in patients with IBS and other FGIDs (functional gastrointestinal disorders), she collaborated with Dr. Peter Gibson at Monash University in Australia to create a more restrictive diet called the low-FODMAP diet. They developed the acronym "FODMAP" when labeling the food components that contribute to digestive symptoms in patients with IBS. These are molecules called short-chain carbohydrates (saccharides) and sugar alcohols (polyols). Dr. Shepherd and Dr. Gibson created this diet—including an elimination phase and a challenge phase—as a way for IBS patients to understand which foods trigger symptoms. When you first start the diet, you will avoid all foods that are high in FODMAPs, and then you will systematically identify which specific FODMAPs are causing your problems.

It is important to note that the final outcome of this elimination diet will be different for everyone. No two people will have the same FODMAP journey, and this is why it is so important to work with a professional to help guide you. Each person will end up with a unique diet pattern that will be the least restrictive with the greatest symptom resolution for them.

fact

There are several sources online with lists for low-FODMAP and high-FODMAP foods. One of the best lists to follow is that of Monash University. You can find comprehensive lists and information at www.fodmaplife .com, and also download the Monash FODMAP Diet app at https://monash fodmap.com/ibs-central/i-have-ibs/ get-the-app/.

Understanding FODMAPs

The acronym "FODMAP" stands for:

- Fermentable
- Oligosaccharides (fructans and galacto-oligosaccharides, a.k.a. GOS)
- Disaccharides (lactose)
- Monosaccharides (excess fructose)
- And
- Polyols (sugar alcohols)

FODMAPs are short-chain carbohydrates (sugars and fibers). Unlike most nutrients, many of these FODMAPs aren't absorbed in the small intestine. Instead, they move along to the large intestine, where gut bacteria use them as a food source. As the bacteria rapidly digest FODMAPs (a process known as fermentation), they produce gases: hydrogen, carbon dioxide, and methane, resulting in gas and bloating. FODMAPs also have an osmotic effect, drawing more fluid into the bowel. In people with IBS and other sensitivities, these gases and fluids contribute to symptoms—otherwise known as unpleasant times! Symptoms can include bloating and distension; diarrhea, constipation, or both; and lower back pain and abdominal pain and pressure.

Some other medical conditions may have symptoms similar to those of IBS, including:

- Celiac disease
- Diverticulitis
- Endometriosis
- Fibromyalgia
- Gallstones
- Inflammatory bowel disease (IBD)
- Pancreatic conditions
- Parasitic infestation
- Thyroid disease
- Tumors of the digestive system

Due to this long list of other possible causes for IBS-like symptoms, health care providers have a chance of incorrectly diagnosing individuals who are experiencing these troubles. Receiving an accurate diagnosis may take time, and that is why it's vital to get as many professional opinions as possible. It is important to be your own medical advocate. Seeking care from a gastroenterologist is a good idea as is asking your primary care doctor about a referral.

Everyone's gut, body chemistry, environment, and stress level are different. So from one person to the next, food can have varying effects. This is why the low-FODMAP diet is so effective: It can be individualized to your particular sensitivities. Through trial and error, the low-FODMAP diet helps you determine what's best for you—and only you. In the following sections you'll learn about the types of FODMAPs, understand which foods they're found in, and discover how they impact your body. As a first step, let's break down the acronym "FODMAP" in more detail.

Fermentable

To put it very simply, fermentation is when a substance is digested by a microorganism. You may be familiar with fermentation in the kitchen (for example, when certain bacteria are added to milk, the fermentation results in yogurt). The *F* in "FODMAP" is about fermentation that happens inside the digestive tract. Trillions of bacteria live in the large intestine, and they help break down food—it's a routine part of digestion. Also normal:

As those bacteria break down (or ferment) food, they release gases. In people *without* IBS, those gases usually don't cause trouble, but, for reasons that aren't completely understood, in those with IBS they contribute to bloating, burping, or flatulence.

Oligosaccharides

Oligosaccharides (including fructans) are a type of carbohydrate. Humans don't have the right enzymes to fully digest them in the small intestine. Instead, they're fermented by bacteria in the large intestine. Because they're such an important food for those gut bacteria, oligosaccharides are sometimes known as prebiotics. They include:

- Fructo-oligosaccharides (called FOS or fructans)—the most common FODMAP to cause symptoms of IBS, found in wheat, rye, onions, garlic, and some fruits, vegetables, beans, and nuts.
- Galacto-oligosaccharides (GOS)— found in dairy products, legumes/beans, and some root vegetables.

---

fact

Although garlic and onions are considered to be high-FODMAP foods, you can still benefit from their flavor in cooking. FODMAPs are water soluble, but they aren't soluble in oil, so you can sauté garlic and onion in oil for a few minutes at the start of a recipe, then discard the solids (and the FODMAPs with them!) and use the flavor-infused oil in your recipe.

Disaccharides

Lactose is a disaccharide—the *D* in FODMAP. Lactose is found in milk, soft cheese, and yogurt. As you probably know, many people have lactose intolerance, a digestive problem also known as lactose malabsorption. People with this condition lack enough of the enzyme lactase, the enzyme that breaks down lactose so that it can be absorbed into the bloodstream. When there's a deficiency in lactase, lactose is instead fermented by gut bacteria, resulting in symptoms. Lactose can also trigger IBS symptoms in people who aren't necessarily deficient in lactase.

Dairy products differ in the amount of lactose that they contain. Therefore, certain dairy products are allowed as part of a low-FODMAP diet. Milk is very high in lactose, so it's wise to seek alternatives or try products like Lactaid or ultrafiltered cow's milk. Soft cheeses are allowed, but only in portions up to 2 ounces. Harder cheeses, such as pecorino, are allowed on the diet because of their lower lactose content. You may want to try lactose-free yogurt and lactose-free cottage cheese as good sources of calcium.

Monosaccharides

Fructose is a monosaccharide—the *M* in "FODMAP." Fructose is a sugar found in many fruits, in honey, and in high fructose corn syrup (HFCS). Fructose malabsorption is experienced in higher rates in those with an FGID or with Crohn's disease.

Fructose malabsorption is the result of fructose not being absorbed well at the level of the small intestine. To digest fructose in the small intestine, the human body uses a transporter called GLUT5. Some people have lower amounts of this transporter, and that results in malabsorption.

Luckily, the extent of the malabsorption is strongly affected by the presence of glucose. When glucose is present, another transporter, known as GLUT2, is activated, which facilitates the absorption of fructose. Therefore, foods that contain equal parts of fructose and glucose (or have more glucose than fructose) can be eaten in moderation without causing symptoms.

This is a strong factor in determining which foods are allowed on the low-FODMAP diet. For example, you might be surprised to see that sugar is allowed in the diet. This is because sugar has equal amounts of fructose and glucose. If you have IBS, foods can be a problem if they contain more than 0.5 grams fructose in excess of glucose per 100-gram serving.

Just remember: If you have fructose malabsorption, you do not need to avoid fructose completely; as long as there is more glucose than fructose in a food, you can eat moderate amounts.

High fructose corn syrup (HFCS), on the other hand, may cause long-term harm. HFCS is an unnatural, industrial food product that you may want to consider steering clear of. HFCS is found in so many processed foods. Here is a short list of where you may find HFCS: beverages, sodas, breads, candy, cake, cereals, barbecue sauce, cookies, cough syrups, yogurt, ice cream, ketchup, marinades, relish, salad dressings, and more.

Polyols

Polyols—the P in "FODMAP"—are sugar alcohols with scientific names that typically end in "ol." Polyols are used as artificial sweeteners and are found naturally in some fruits and vegetables, such as cauliflower, mushrooms, blackberries, and more. Polyol types include:

- Isomalt
- Maltitol
- Mannitol
- Polydextrose
- Sorbitol
- Xylitol

Polyol malabsorption is a fairly common condition. In addition to contributing to excessive intestinal gas and bloating, polyols are also strong contributors to diarrhea, due to their laxative effect. As you follow the low-FODMAP diet, you will become very good at reading ingredients labels and looking for the presence of polyol artificial sweeteners. Watch out for anything that's labeled as sugar-free or has sugar alcohols (often ending in "ol") in the ingredients list. These polyols can cause symptoms for people with digestive disorders if they contain more than 0.4 grams of polyols per serving.

Who Can Benefit from a Low-FODMAP Diet?

The low-FODMAP diet was designed to offer patients with IBS a way of eating that does not aggravate symptoms. The diet also seems to help people with other functional gastrointestinal disorders (FGIDs), SIBO (small intestinal bacterial overgrowth), GERD (gastroesophageal reflux disease), celiac disease, and gluten intolerance. It does not necessarily "cure" the underlying problem, but it has been shown to be effective in reducing abdominal pain, bloating, flatulence, constipation, and diarrhea.

If you've been suffering from intestinal pain or discomfort and think the cause may be one of these conditions, it would be helpful to learn more about them so you know the right questions to ask your doctor or gastroenterologist at your next appointment.

IBS

Doctors have a set of diagnostic criteria called the Rome IV criteria for making a firm diagnosis of IBS. The Rome criteria require that a person experience abdominal pain or discomfort, along with a marked change in bowel habits, with symptom onset at least six months prior to diagnosis. In addition, they should have recurrent abdominal pain on the average of at least one day a week in the last three months, associated with two or more of the following criteria:

- Pain is related to defecation
- Pain is associated with a change in frequency of stool
- Pain is associated with a change in form (appearance) of stool

In the real world, doctors tend to give the diagnosis to anyone who has chronic digestive symptoms without any identifiable reason, regardless of whether or not the symptoms meet the Rome IV criteria.

The diagnosis of IBS is based on the symptoms a patient reports and is made after ruling out other disorders. Typically, your doctor will conduct a comprehensive physical exam, order blood work, and ask you for a stool sample to look for the presence of rectal bleeding. Depending on your symptom picture, the doctor may recommend that you undergo further testing, such as a colonoscopy or an endoscopy. These tests are not positive indicators of IBS, but rather are used to rule out other possible reasons for your symptoms.

Food Allergy or Intolerance

A food allergy is an immune system reaction to a particular food. When a person has a food allergy, eating even a small amount of the offending food will prompt the immune system to release chemicals that cause a variety of symptoms. You are probably familiar with typical allergy symptoms—hives, itching, and lip swelling—in addition to the more serious symptoms of difficulty breathing and swelling of the throat. Food allergies can also create gastrointestinal symptoms such as vomiting, diarrhea, and/or abdominal pain. The most common food allergens include eggs, fish and shellfish, milk, peanuts, soy, tree nuts, and wheat.

In an allergic reaction, the body perceives a food as an invader, and as a result it releases an antibody known as immunoglobulin E, or IgE. The IgE then triggers the release of histamine and other chemicals, causing allergy symptoms. IgE release can be identified through the use of allergy tests, thus helping to confirm a diagnosis of a food allergy.

A food intolerance, also known as a food sensitivity, is a different type of negative reaction to a food. An allergy involves a reaction on the part of the immune system (with an IgE response), while a food intolerance is a reaction on the part of the gastrointestinal system (although there may still be some immune system involvement). Therefore, symptoms of a food intolerance are often gastrointestinal in nature.

Celiac Disease

Celiac disease is an autoimmune condition in which the body's immune system reacts to the presence of gluten. Gluten is a protein found in barley, rye, and wheat. When a person with celiac disease eats something containing gluten, the immune system attacks and damages the villi lining the small intestine. The damage to the villi prevents the body from being able to absorb important nutrients. This can result in serious health problems and a wide variety of symptoms. Celiac disease is diagnosed with initial blood screening, followed by an endoscopy with a biopsy of the lining of the small intestine.

The gastrointestinal symptoms of celiac disease are very similar to those of IBS: abdominal pain, bloating, and diarrhea. Research indicates that, compared to the population at large, people who've been diagnosed with IBS are four times more likely to have celiac disease. So if you have IBS, it is essential that you be screened for celiac disease before beginning the low-FODMAP diet or any gluten-free diet. People with celiac disease must follow a strict, lifelong gluten-free diet.

Gluten Intolerance

When a person who *doesn't* have celiac disease reacts negatively to foods containing gluten, it's known as gluten intolerance or non-celiac gluten sensitivity (NCGS). Unlike with celiac disease, with a gluten intolerance (NCGS) the immune system doesn't attack the villi, so there's no concern about damage to the small intestine. Therefore, a person with gluten intolerance can eat gluten without the concern of permanent damage, but they may suffer the consequence of undesirable symptoms.

The symptoms of gluten intolerance may be gastrointestinal in nature, with symptoms such as abdominal pain, constipation, and diarrhea. There is also the theory that a gluten intolerance may cause other symptoms throughout the body—symptoms such as brain fog, fatigue, headaches, and joint pain. Like other intolerances, a gluten intolerance is typically identified through the use of an elimination diet and challenge test.

> **question**
>
> **Will the Diet Work for Me?**
> The low-FODMAP dietary approach has been shown to help between 50 and 75 percent of people with IBS who follow the diet carefully with a dietitian's guidance.

The Elimination and Challenge Phases

This diet has an elimination phase and a challenge phase. In the elimination phase, you'll strictly avoid all high-FODMAP foods for two to six weeks. Most people who try the low-FODMAP diet see significant improvement in their symptoms by the four-week mark, but you may find that you feel better even sooner. However, don't despair if it takes longer for you to see improvement—everyone's body is unique and will be affected differently by the diet.

Throughout the elimination and challenge phases, be sure to use a food and symptom diary. You can create your own symptom diary using the following template or one you find online. This valuable resource will help you and your doctor and registered dietitian to pinpoint your triggers.

During the challenge phase (or reintroduction phase) you will detect personal triggers by reintroducing one FODMAP category at a time, one food at a time. The timing of the challenge phase will depend on how you're feeling and how quickly your body responds to the absence of problem foods. If you're feeling significantly better one week into the elimination phase, you might be able to start the challenge phase after two weeks.

After the challenge phase, FODMAPs that do not trigger symptoms can be a part of your regular diet again, and some

DAILY SYMPTOM DIARY

Date	Foods eaten	Portion sizes	Other factors	Symptoms
Breakfast				
Snack				
Lunch				
Snack				
Dinner				
Dessert/Snack				

FODMAPs may be tolerated in limited portions. It's important to finish the challenge phase so you can enjoy a varied diet full of the essential nutrients from the vitamins and minerals found in fruits, vegetables, legumes, nuts, seeds, healthy fats, and protein. You need these foods in order to maintain your health.

> **fact**
>
> For some people, in the long term, a certain level of FODMAP restriction may be necessary to regulate symptoms. It is never suggested to follow the low-FODMAP diet for life.

As an example, if you follow the diet correctly, the challenge phase may show you that polyols don't cause an issue for your gut. If you were to stay in the elimination phase for a long time without trying the challenge phase, you'd miss out on the health benefits of foods such as cauliflower, mushrooms, snow peas, apples, apricots, Asian pears, blackberries, nectarines, peaches, pears, plums, prunes, and watermelon, which are all high in polyols but (depending on which other FODMAPs you're sensitive to) may be okay for you to eat whole or in specific serving sizes.

Elimination Phase Overview

The elimination phase of the diet typically lasts two to six weeks. Without argument, this is certainly the strictest phase of the diet. Many foods that you have typically eaten will now be off-limits. But don't worry; although you will have to change the way you eat, you will still be able to eat lots of delicious foods! Also, you'll find that there are many substitutes you can use so you can still enjoy your favorite recipes.

You can make the decision about how long to stick to the elimination phase with the help of your physician or your registered dietitian. The timing will depend on how you're feeling and how quickly your body responds to the absence of problem foods. Your doctor or registered dietitian will provide you with a list of foods you will need to refrain from during the elimination phase.

Challenge Phase Overview

In this phase, you will gradually expand the number of foods you eat. You will do this by reintroducing foods into your diet, one FODMAP group at a time. As you do this, you'll gain a better awareness of which foods contain which FODMAPs and which FODMAPs your body is able to tolerate. After you complete the diet, you will be able to eat more of your favorite foods with confidence.

You will spend approximately one week reintroducing each FODMAP type, starting with the smallest dose on a Monday and gradually increasing throughout the week.

The order in which you introduce each type of FODMAP is up to you. However, fructans and GOS should be saved for last, as they are not absorbed in *anyone's* small intestine and are therefore the most likely to cause symptoms.

If you don't experience a return of your digestive symptoms after introducing a new food, you can conclude that your body can tolerate that food and other foods from that FODMAP group. Make note of this in your symptom diary. If your symptoms return in response to a reintroduced food, eliminate that FODMAP group again until you feel better. If you experience a severe reaction to the small Monday dose, you don't need to continue eating that food all week—it's okay to conclude that you have a sensitivity to that FODMAP.

How to Read Food Labels

Properly reading food labels will help ensure success with the low-FODMAP diet. Food labels list ingredients in descending order of weight; the ingredients that make up the greatest portion of the product's weight are listed first. For many people, some FODMAPs are an issue only when consumed regularly and in significant amounts. If a high-FODMAP food is listed on an ingredients list but is present in small amounts (such as when the label indicates the ingredient is less than 2%), it most likely will be suitable to consume.

When first starting the diet, it will take some time to learn how to read labels. Rest assured that with each trip to the grocery store, your confidence will improve and time spent researching will decrease. You can improve your experience of shopping by finding a low-FODMAP grocery list online, or by using a low-FODMAP app such as Monash University's, to quickly look up any foods and serving sizes you're uncertain about.

Of course, you can avoid long ingredients lists entirely by choosing whole foods, such as low-FODMAP fruits, vegetables, nuts, grains, and seeds, as well as lean proteins and lactose-free dairy products.

> **alert**
>
> Steer clear of breads, cereals, biscuits, pastas, and other products whose labels list wheat or rye as a main ingredient (anywhere from first to third on the ingredients list).

Some foods that are low in FODMAPs might still be troublesome:

- All meats and animal proteins are low in FODMAPs (unless they are processed with high-FODMAP ingredients); however, fatty meats take a much longer time to digest than lean meats, and this can cause diarrhea. As an example, fruit takes about a half hour to digest, while fatty meat can take days. It's wise to choose lean meats on the low-FODMAP diet, because it means easier digestion and a more peaceful gut.

- Broccoli and kale are cruciferous vegetables and may cause gas due to their content of raffinose, an indigestible sugar.
- Eggs that have been boiled can cause symptoms in people who have egg intolerance—in other words, who don't have the right enzymes to break down the egg's proteins.
- Potatoes, corn, and other starchy vegetables can produce gas in the large intestine.
- Oat products (such as oatmeal, oatmeal cookies, and oat bran) can all result in excessive gas because of their high soluble-fiber content. Quick-cooking oats are okay on the diet at a ¼-cup serving size.

A Word on Wheat and Gluten

The low-FODMAP diet is not a gluten-free diet, but it's a diet that avoids foods high in fructans, which fall under the O in "FODMAPs," oligosaccharides. Wheat contains fructans and also gluten, but gluten itself does not contain fructans. The diet can be confusing sometimes, because several gluten-free products work on the low-FODMAP diet, but not all low-FODMAP foods are gluten-free. So let's discuss some of the reasons wheat can cause digestive issues for various people.

People with celiac disease and other forms of gluten sensitivity (refer to the Gluten Intolerance section in this chapter for more information) need to avoid gluten. They must use caution when abiding by the low-FODMAP diet, because some low-FODMAP foods contain gluten. For example, ½ cup of cooked wheat pasta is low in FODMAPs (fructans), but it also has gluten, so it's okay on the low-FODMAP diet, but it's off-limits for those avoiding gluten. Oats are gluten-free *and* allowed on the low-FODMAP diet in certain quantities; however, someone with celiac disease or a gluten sensitivity may choose to buy gluten-free oats to avoid the risk of the oats being cross-contaminated with wheat during processing. Thankfully, gluten-free products made at 100 percent gluten-free facilities are more widely available today than they've ever been before.

The specific compound that causes trouble for people with celiac disease is a protein called gliadin. It's a component of gluten, which of course is found in a wide variety of foods and ingredients. For someone with celiac disease, ingesting *any* amount of gluten can cause uncomfortable or painful symptoms and long-term health problems.

For people who don't have celiac disease but do have IBS, gliadin isn't a problem, and neither is gluten itself. Instead, trouble is caused by another component of wheat: fructans. Of all the FODMAPs, fructans are the most common trigger for IBS symptoms. Many sources of gluten in a typical Western diet—wheat, barley, and rye—contain fructans as well. That's why many gluten-free products work well for low-FODMAP eating. However, gluten-free isn't the *same* as fructan-free, because fructans are found in many other common ingredients, including onions, garlic, and many beans and nuts.

essential

More doctors are prescribing gluten-free diets to patients with non-celiac autoimmune diseases to help combat inflammation and oxidative stress. However, there is still a lack of evidence-based information about dietary treatments for autoimmune diseases.

On the low-FODMAP diet, you avoid (among other things) wheat, barley, and rye in order to avoid a specific kind of carbohydrate in those grains (fructans). You aren't intentionally avoiding the gluten protein gliadin, as people with celiac disease and gluten sensitivity need to. Therefore, on the low-FODMAP diet, it's acceptable to eat foods that contain gluten but are low in FODMAPs. One example is spelt sourdough bread—it's suitable on the diet at two slices per serving (remember to abide by serving sizes to keep the FODMAP content in acceptable range).

CHAPTER 2

Basics from Scratch

Easy Onion- and Garlic-Free Chicken Stock

This is a great low-FODMAP staple to have ready for soups, sauces, rice, and other low-FODMAP dishes included in this book. You can use fresh rosemary and thyme (rather than dried) if you prefer; just use about three times the quantity called for, since the flavor in fresh herbs is less concentrated.

Makes 2 quarts

Per Serving
(Serving size: 1 cup)

Calories	20
Fat	1g
Protein	4g
Sodium	10mg
Fiber	0g
Carbohydrates	0g
Sugar	0g

1 (2-pound) rotisserie chicken

2 quarts cold water

2 medium carrots, peeled and cut into chunks

1 medium stalk celery with leaves, cut into chunks

1 large stalk bok choy, cut into chunks

½ teaspoon dried rosemary

½ teaspoon dried thyme

4 sprigs parsley

2 bay leaves

8 whole peppercorns

1. Remove meat from rotisserie chicken and set aside to use for other recipes. Place chicken carcass and water in a 4- to 6-quart slow cooker; arrange as needed to make sure carcass is fully covered with water.
2. Add vegetables, herbs, and peppercorns to slow cooker. Set temperature to low, and cook 6–8 hours.
3. Use tongs to transfer chicken bones from slow cooker and discard. Place a large sieve over a large bowl. Drain contents from slow cooker through sieve. Discard large vegetable pieces, bay leaves, and peppercorns. Use a large spoon to skim fat from surface of stock.
4. Cool stock completely, pour into glass jars or plastic containers, and refrigerate up to 1 week or freeze up to 3 months.

Vegetable Stock

Use this as a base for low-FODMAP soups and other recipes, especially for vegetarian and vegan dishes.

1 tablespoon garlic-infused olive oil

½ medium stalk celery, cut into chunks

2 medium stalks bok choy, cut into chunks

2 large carrots, peeled and cut into chunks

1 small bulb fennel, cut into chunks

4 quarts cold water

6 sprigs flat-leaf parsley

1 bay leaf

1 teaspoon whole black peppercorns

Makes 2 quarts
Per Serving (Serving size: 1 cup)
Calories 20
Fat 2g
Protein 0g
Sodium 16mg
Fiber 0g
Carbohydrates 1g
Sugar 0g

1. Heat oil in a large stockpot over medium-high heat. Add celery, bok choy, carrots, and fennel and cook, stirring occasionally until vegetables begin to soften, 5–7 minutes.
2. Add water, parsley, bay leaf, and peppercorns. Bring to a boil, then reduce heat to low and simmer until stock is reduced by half, 1–1½ hours.
3. Strain stock through a fine-mesh sieve into a large bowl, discarding vegetables, bay leaf, and peppercorns. Store in an airtight container in refrigerator 4–5 days or in freezer 4–6 months.

Basic Mayonnaise

It can sometimes be hard to find low-FODMAP mayonnaise, but it's easy to make your own at home. If you can't find safflower oil for this recipe, you can use sunflower oil instead.

Makes 2 cups
Per Serving
(Serving size: 1 tablespoon)
Calories 86
Fat 9g
Protein 0g
Sodium 46mg
Fiber 0g
Carbohydrates 0g
Sugar 0g

2 large eggs

2 tablespoons Dijon mustard

1⅓ cups safflower oil

2 tablespoons fresh lemon juice

¼ teaspoon salt

¼ teaspoon ground black pepper

1. In a food processor fitted with a blade attachment, combine eggs and mustard. Process until evenly combined.
2. Keep food processor running and add oil in a slow stream until completely combined.
3. Add lemon juice, salt, and pepper, and pulse until smooth. Store in a jar or container with a tight-fitting lid in refrigerator up to 3 days.

Sweet Barbecue Sauce

Most barbecue sauces at your local supermarket are filled with high-FODMAP ingredients such as high fructose corn syrup, onions, and garlic. In order to keep enjoying barbecue sauce, you will need to make your own. For a smokier barbecue sauce, you can add specialty ingredients such as smoked sea salt or smoked paprika to this base recipe.

1 cup Tomato Purée (see recipe in this chapter)

1 tablespoon Dijon mustard

1 tablespoon blackstrap molasses

1½ tablespoons pure maple syrup

½ teaspoon ground cinnamon

½ teaspoon ground cumin

½ teaspoon dried oregano

½ teaspoon white wine vinegar

½ teaspoon arrowroot powder

½ teaspoon paprika

⅛ teaspoon ground red pepper

⅛ teaspoon ground nutmeg

⅛ teaspoon sea salt

Makes 1 cup	
Per Serving **(Serving size: 2 tablespoons)**	
Calories	40
Fat	1g
Protein	1g
Sodium	192mg
Fiber	1g
Carbohydrates	7g
Sugar	5g

In a small saucepan over medium-high heat, bring all ingredients just to a boil. Lower heat and simmer, uncovered, 5–10 minutes or until sauce thickens.

Aioli

Typical aioli is garlic-based, but this low-FODMAP version will give you all the flavor with none of the dietary troubles. This aioli tastes delicious spread on sandwiches or burgers or used as a dip for appetizers.

Makes 1¼ cups	
Per Serving	
(Serving size: 1 tablespoon)	
Calories	99
Fat	11g
Protein	0g
Sodium	34mg
Fiber	0g
Carbohydrates	0g
Sugar	0g

1 teaspoon Dijon mustard

1 large egg

¼ cup garlic-infused olive oil

¾ cup olive oil

2 teaspoons fresh lemon juice

¼ teaspoon kosher salt

⅛ teaspoon ground black pepper

1. Place mustard and egg in the bowl of a food processor fitted with a blade attachment.
2. With the motor running, slowly add garlic-infused oil, followed by olive oil, until completely combined, about 2 minutes.
3. Stop processor, add lemon juice, salt, and pepper, and pulse until thoroughly mixed. If necessary, stop and scrape down the sides of the bowl using a rubber spatula, then continue to pulse until well combined.
4. Let aioli sit 30 minutes before using. Refrigerate in a container with a tight-fitting lid up to 3 days.

Tomato Purée

Due to the concern about excessive fructose in canned tomato purée, it's a good idea to make your own. This is a basic recipe, but feel free to experiment with other FODMAP-friendly seasonings, such as basil, oregano, or parsley.

1 tablespoon garlic-infused olive oil

5 medium ripe tomatoes, cored, seeded, and diced

1 teaspoon sea salt

¼ teaspoon ground black pepper

1. Heat oil over medium-low heat in a large saucepan. Add tomatoes and stir. Season with salt and pepper. Sauté, stirring occasionally, 15–20 minutes or until tomatoes are soft and broken down. Remove from heat and let cool.
2. Transfer cooled tomatoes to a food processor and blend completely. Set a large strainer over a large bowl and strain mixture. Press down with a large spoon to completely separate solids in strainer from purée in bowl.
3. Transfer to an airtight container and store in refrigerator 5–7 days or in freezer 3–4 months.

Makes 1½ cups

Per Serving
(Serving size: ¼ cup)

Calories	34
Fat	2g
Protein	1g
Sodium	238mg
Fiber	1g
Carbohydrates	3g
Sugar	2g

Make Your Own Tomato Paste

You can also use this tomato purée to make tomato paste. Simply pour 1½ cups tomato purée into an ovenproof skillet. Bake, uncovered, at 300°F for about 2 hours, stirring every 20 minutes until purée thickens to a paste-like consistency. Let cool completely before using. Makes ⅓ cup. Store any unused paste in an airtight container in the refrigerator for up to 3 days or in the freezer for several months.

Basic Marinara Sauce

If you've been following the low-FODMAP diet, you know most marinara and pasta sauces are made with high-FODMAP ingredients such as onions and garlic. This sauce is a lifesaver! If you prefer using canned tomatoes rather than fresh ones, you can replace the Romas with a 35-ounce can of San Marzano tomatoes.

Makes 4¼ cups	
Per Serving (Serving size: ¼ cup)	
Calories	29
Fat	2g
Protein	1g
Sodium	139mg
Fiber	1g
Carbohydrates	2g
Sugar	2g

Canned Tomatoes and the Low-FODMAP Diet

Although tomatoes are allowed on the low-FODMAP diet, this does not mean that all tomato products are okay. For example, canned tomato paste and purée may have excessive levels of fructose. It is best to use fresh tomatoes or canned tomatoes with thin, watery juice.

16 medium Roma tomatoes, chopped

1 tablespoon garlic-infused olive oil

1 tablespoon plus 2 teaspoons extra-virgin olive oil

¼ teaspoon red pepper flakes

1 teaspoon salt

20 basil leaves, chopped

1. Add tomatoes to a large mixing bowl. Using your hands or a potato masher, crush tomatoes and break up into small pieces.
2. Heat a 2-quart pot over medium-high heat. Pour oils into pot, and stir in red pepper flakes. Wait 1 minute, then add crushed tomatoes and stir well.
3. Increase heat to high and sprinkle in salt. Add basil and stir to combine.
4. Bring sauce to a boil and cover. Reduce heat to medium-high and cook 10–12 minutes, keeping sauce at a rolling simmer.
5. Uncover and cook another 5 minutes. Remove from heat. Use immediately, or transfer to an airtight container and store in refrigerator 3–4 days or in freezer 5–6 months.

Tartar Sauce

This low-FODMAP sauce pairs well with fish and shellfish recipes like the ones in Chapter 6.

3 tablespoons Basic Mayonnaise (see recipe in this chapter)

3 tablespoons lactose-free plain yogurt

1/16 teaspoon wheat-free asafetida powder

1 tablespoon relish

1 teaspoon granulated sugar

Add all ingredients to a small bowl. Stir well with a spoon. Store in refrigerator in a container with a tight-fitting lid up to 3 days.

Makes ½ cup

Per Serving
(Serving size: 1 tablespoon)

Calories	44
Fat	4g
Protein	0g
Sodium	40mg
Fiber	0g
Carbohydrates	2g
Sugar	2g

Asafetida Powder

Asafetida (also known as asafoetida or hing) is used often in Indian vegetarian cooking. It's derived from a species of giant fennel and has a unique smell and powerful flavor. It is suitable for the low-FODMAP diet as an onion and garlic replacement. Make sure you buy a wheat-free version, and try just a little bit at a time and adjust the amount accordingly—using too much can ruin your dish.

Flax Eggs

Add this egg replacement mixture to recipes calling for 1 large egg. You can purchase ground flaxseed meal or grind your own at home in a blender.

Makes 1 "egg"
Per Serving (Serving size: 1 "egg")
Calories 35
Fat 2g
Protein 2g
Sodium 0mg
Fiber 2g
Carbohydrates 2g
Sugar 0g

1 tablespoon flaxseed meal

3 tablespoons water

Combine flaxseed meal and water in a small bowl and allow to sit 5 minutes.

Gluten-Free All-Purpose 1-to-1 Flour

Use this gluten-free flour to make sandwich breads, pancake mix, crepes, waffles, pie crust, and more.

Makes 11½ cups
Per Serving (Serving size: ¼ cup)
Calories 141
Fat 0g
Protein 2g
Sodium 4mg
Fiber 2g
Carbohydrates 32g
Sugar 0g

3 cups sweet white rice flour

3 cups brown rice flour

3 cups white rice flour

2½ cups tapioca flour/starch

2½ tablespoons xanthan gum

In a large bowl, whisk all ingredients together until well combined. Store in an airtight container.

Gluten-Free Bread Flour 1

If your supermarket's freezer isn't stocked with gluten-free bread, or if you just feel like baking, use this mix as a base to then add yeast, salt, and other ingredients.

1 cup millet flour

1 cup sorghum flour

1 cup potato flour

2 cups rice flour

Place all ingredients in a large container with a lid. Stir to combine, or cover and shake. Store in refrigerator for freshness. Allow to come to room temperature before using.

Makes 5 cups

Per Serving
(Serving size: 1/4 cup)

Calories	137
Fat	1g
Protein	3g
Sodium	4mg
Fiber	1g
Carbohydrates	30g
Sugar	0g

Gluten-Free Bread Tip

Using high-protein flours such as millet and sorghum adds structure and flavor to bread, so these are key ingredients when you're leaving out the gluten.

Gluten-Free Bread Flour 2

Brown rice flour has a neutral flavor and adds stability to this mixture, while sorghum flour provides the protein structure for the bread.

Makes 3 cups	
Per Serving **(Serving size: ¼ cup)**	
Calories	132
Fat	1g
Protein	2g
Sodium	1mg
Fiber	1g
Carbohydrates	30g
Sugar	0g

1¼ cups brown rice flour

¾ cup potato starch

½ cup tapioca flour/starch

½ cup sorghum flour

Place all ingredients in a large container with a lid. Stir to combine, or cover and shake. Store in refrigerator for freshness. Allow to come to room temperature before using.

Gluten-Free Pizza Dough

Try making your own dough at home, and get creative with your pizza! There are many low-FODMAP topping possibilities, so this is a dish you can have over and over again without getting bored.

1 cup warm water

1 teaspoon light brown sugar

1 tablespoon active dry yeast

2½ cups gluten-free all-purpose flour

¼ teaspoon gluten-free baking powder

¾ teaspoon salt

2½ tablespoons olive oil, divided

Makes 1 crust

Per Serving
(Serving size: ⅛ crust)

Calories	222
Fat	4g
Protein	2g
Sodium	233mg
Fiber	0g
Carbohydrates	41g
Sugar	1g

1. In a small glass bowl, mix water, sugar, and yeast.
2. In the bowl of a stand mixer, combine flour, baking powder, and salt.
3. Add yeast mixture to bowl and, with dough hook attachment, mix on medium speed. Slowly add 1½ tablespoons oil, and continue mixing until dough forms a mass that pulls away from the side of the bowl.
4. Grease dough with remaining 1 tablespoon oil, transfer to a medium bowl, cover with a towel, and allow to rise in a warm area until doubled in size, about 1½ hours.
5. When ready to make pizza, prebake crust at 350°F 25–30 minutes. Remove from oven and add toppings. Bake 15–20 more minutes or until toppings are warmed through. Serve.

Vegan Parmesan Cheez

Many vegan cheeses are made with cashews, which are high in FODMAPs. Brazil nuts provide a nice consistency and earthiness that make this cheese a winner to sprinkle on your favorite vegan dishes. (As a precaution you should avoid eating a large amount of Brazil nuts multiple days in a row due to their high selenium content.)

Makes 1 cup

Per Serving
(Serving size: 1 tablespoon)

Calories	42
Fat	4g
Protein	1g
Sodium	25mg
Fiber	1g
Carbohydrates	1g
Sugar	0g

What Is Nutritional Yeast?

Often found in vegan dishes, nutritional yeast is a deactivated yeast used as a seasoning, known for its cheesy, nutty flavor and rich nutritional profile. It's a popular plant-based source of B vitamins, including B_{12}. It can be found at most grocery stores, often in the baking aisle or among the spices and seasonings.

¾ cup Brazil nuts

¼ teaspoon sea salt

1 tablespoon nutritional yeast

1 tablespoon chopped flat-leaf parsley

1 tablespoon fresh lemon juice

1. Preheat oven to 275°F. Line a baking sheet with parchment paper.
2. Process nuts in a food processor until just crumbly. Place in a medium bowl and add salt, nutritional yeast, parsley, and lemon juice. Stir well until combined. Spread mixture on a baking sheet.
3. Bake 35–40 minutes, tossing at least three times during baking, until golden around edges.
4. Remove from oven and allow to cool. May be refrigerated in an airtight container up to 2 months.

CHAPTER 3

Breakfast and Brunch

Autumn Chia Breakfast Bowl

When the cool of autumn starts to roll in, warm up with this healthy and hearty breakfast bowl. The chia seeds and oats in this bowl will help keep you feeling full and satisfied all morning long.

Serves 2

Per Serving

Calories 531
Fat 19g
Protein 20g
Sodium 324mg
Fiber 18g
Carbohydrates 72g
Sugar 4g

3 cups water

¼ teaspoon salt

1 cup steel cut oats

½ cup lactose-free milk

3 tablespoons chia seeds

1 tablespoon halved macadamia nuts

1 tablespoon sliced almonds

½ teaspoon ground cinnamon

1 tablespoon no-sugar-added dried cranberries

1. In a medium saucepan, bring water and salt to a boil, then add oats. Add milk and stir.
2. Add chia seeds, macadamia nuts, almonds, cinnamon, and cranberries, and stir again.
3. Cover and cook 15–20 minutes, stirring occasionally, until chia seeds become soft and gel-like. Serve immediately.

Cinnamon Spice Granola

Due to their high fiber content, larger servings of oats may cause intestinal gas for people with IBS, so be sure to stick with a ¼-cup serving (measured dry) of quick-cooking oats. This granola tastes great mixed with lactose-free yogurt.

2 cups quick-cooking oats

1 cup walnut pieces

1 teaspoon ground cinnamon

½ teaspoon ground nutmeg

¼ teaspoon ground cloves

3 tablespoons light brown sugar

¼ cup pure maple syrup

¼ cup safflower oil

Serves 8	
Per Serving	
Calories	281
Fat	17g
Protein	5g
Sodium	4mg
Fiber	3g
Carbohydrates	28g
Sugar	12g

1. Preheat oven to 350°F.
2. Combine all ingredients in a large bowl.
3. Spread mixture in an even layer on a baking sheet and bake 20 minutes. Stir once halfway through the cooking time.
4. Allow to cool before serving.

Tomato Spinach Frittata Muffins

Enjoy frittatas in a whole new way with these muffins. They're easy to make and fun to bake, and they're a great make-ahead breakfast!

Serves 12

Per Serving

Calories 82
Fat 5g
Protein 7g
Sodium 146mg
Fiber 0g
Carbohydrates 2g
Sugar 1g

You Can Eat the Green!

Whole onions, shallots, and the white parts of green onions (a.k.a. scallions) are high in FODMAPs. They contain fructans—which are oligosaccharides (the *O* in FODMAPs). The *green* parts of green onions, however, are low in FODMAPs and are safe to eat on the low-FODMAP diet.

2 cups finely chopped spinach

1½ cups chopped tomatoes

1 green onion, finely chopped, green parts only

½ cup crumbled feta cheese

10 large eggs

2 tablespoons lactose-free milk

1 teaspoon dried oregano

⅛ teaspoon salt

¼ teaspoon ground black pepper

1. Preheat oven to 375°F. Grease a twelve-cup muffin pan with cooking spray.
2. Distribute spinach, tomatoes, green onions, and feta evenly among muffin cups.
3. In a medium bowl, whisk together eggs, milk, oregano, salt, and pepper. Pour egg mixture evenly into each muffin cup.
4. Bake 15–20 minutes or until eggs are completely set. Serve.

Flourless Vegan Banana Peanut Butter Pancakes

You're sure to love these easy and nutritious pancakes. You'll never even know they're vegan!

2 Flax Eggs (Chapter 2)

½ medium ripe banana

1 teaspoon chia seeds

1 tablespoon peanut butter

1 tablespoon coconut oil

Serves 1	
Per Serving	
Calories	363
Fat	27g
Protein	8g
Sodium	0mg
Fiber	7g
Carbohydrates	22g
Sugar	8g

1. In a glass measuring cup, mix together Flax Eggs, banana, chia seeds, and peanut butter. Be sure to mash bananas well, or use an immersion blender to mix ingredients on low speed until smooth.
2. Heat oil in a medium skillet over medium heat. Pour batter onto the skillet in two puddles, and cook pancakes until bubbly on top and golden on bottom, about 4 minutes. Flip and cook about 2 more minutes. Serve.

Passion Fruit Smoothie Bowl

Passion fruit is a sweet and tart fruit that does well when paired with other sweet ingredients. It is often used in drinks, sorbet, tartlets, cakes, bread, and more. In this breakfast bowl it brightens up the flavors and gives the whole dish a tropical feel.

Serves 1	
Per Serving	
Calories	365
Fat	19g
Protein	13g
Sodium	245mg
Fiber	11g
Carbohydrates	39g
Sugar	20g

Toasting Coconut

To toast coconut, place shredded coconut in a small skillet and heat over medium-high heat. Stir frequently until flakes become golden brown. Remove from heat and set aside. You can also toast coconut in an oven. Heat oven to 350°F. Spread coconut evenly on a rimmed baking sheet, and bake for 8 minutes or until light golden brown, stirring occasionally.

½ medium banana, frozen

1 tablespoon chia seeds

½ cup lactose-free vanilla yogurt

½ teaspoon alcohol-free vanilla extract

1 cup unsweetened almond milk

½ cup ice

Pulp of ½ medium passion fruit

1 tablespoon almond butter

1 tablespoon shredded unsweetened coconut, toasted

1. Blend banana, chia seeds, yogurt, vanilla, almond milk, and ice in a blender until smooth.
2. Pour into a serving bowl and top with passion fruit, almond butter, and toasted coconut. Serve.

Eggs Baked in Heirloom Tomatoes

As you cut into these juicy tomatoes, savor the aroma of herbs and the warm, baked gooeyness of the egg and cheese. If you don't have heirloom tomatoes, choose other large fresh tomatoes that have nice, thick skins.

4 large, round heirloom tomatoes

3 tablespoons olive oil

½ teaspoon herbes de Provence

¼ teaspoon salt

1 teaspoon ground black pepper

4 large eggs

¼ cup grated Parmesan cheese

¼ cup crumbled feta cheese

2 teaspoons lactose-free milk

Serves 4	
Per Serving	
Calories	239
Fat	18g
Protein	11g
Sodium	422mg
Fiber	2g
Carbohydrates	7g
Sugar	4g

1. Preheat oven to 375°F.
2. Slice off tops of tomatoes, and use a paring knife or small spoon to gently remove cores and seeds, making sure not to pierce bottoms of tomatoes but cutting enough flesh to leave ample space to drop in egg.
3. Arrange tomatoes so they are snug in an 8" × 8" or larger baking dish lightly greased with cooking spray. Drizzle each tomato with ¼ of the oil, and then sprinkle evenly with herbes de Provence, salt, and pepper.
4. Crack an egg into each tomato. Top each evenly with Parmesan, feta, and milk.
5. Bake 20 minutes for runny eggs and 30 minutes or more for harder yolks. Serve.

Eggs with Spinach and Chickpeas

Shake up your morning and try something different with your eggs—like combining them with high-protein chickpeas. You'll love the flavors of this healthy and filling dish!

Serves 2

Per Serving

Calories 551
Fat 39g
Protein 16g
Sodium 1,178mg
Fiber 9g
Carbohydrates 34g
Sugar 12g

Canned Chickpeas Are Allowed?

Canning allows the GOS in chickpeas to leach out into the water of the can, making them lower in FODMAPs than freshly cooked chickpeas. So they're low in FODMAPs as long as you rinse and drain them and stick with a ¼-cup serving.

4 tablespoons olive oil, divided

4 cups coarsely chopped baby spinach

⅛ teaspoon wheat-free asafetida powder

½ teaspoon salt

½ teaspoon ground black pepper

¼ teaspoon smoked paprika

½ cup canned chickpeas, rinsed and drained

2½ cups canned whole San Marzano tomatoes, crushed

3½ cups Vegetable Stock (Chapter 2), divided

2 large eggs

¼ cup crumbled goat cheese

1. Heat 1 tablespoon oil in a large, heavy pan or cast iron skillet over medium heat. Add spinach, asafetida, salt, and pepper. Cook until spinach is slightly wilted, about 2–3 minutes. Transfer to a medium bowl and set aside.
2. Using the same pan, heat 2 tablespoons oil over medium heat. Add paprika, chickpeas, and tomatoes, and stir. Cook 10 minutes.
3. Add 3 cups stock and bring to a boil. Reduce heat to medium and simmer until sauce is thickened, 15–20 minutes. Add spinach and remaining ½ cup stock and simmer 8–10 minutes.
4. Heat remaining 1 tablespoon oil in an 8-inch nonstick skillet over medium-high heat. Crack both eggs into skillet and fry sunny side up until edges are crispy, about 2–3 minutes.
5. Place chickpea mixture in serving bowls, and top each with a fried egg and goat cheese. Serve.

Breakfast Tacos

These tacos make a satisfying and delicious breakfast and come together in no time. They are easy to eat at home or on the go, and the whole family will love this protein-packed breakfast!

4 large eggs

4 large egg whites

¼ cup lactose-free milk

1 tablespoon chopped cilantro

¼ teaspoon salt

½ teaspoon ground black pepper

4 strips bacon

¼ cup diced green bell pepper

¼ teaspoon ground cumin

4 (8-inch) soft corn tortillas

½ cup shredded Cheddar cheese

¼ cup lactose-free sour cream

¼ cup salsa

Serves 4	
Per Serving	
Calories	293
Fat	2g
Protein	20g
Sodium	698mg
Fiber	2g
Carbohydrates	15g
Sugar	4g

1. In a medium bowl, combine eggs, egg whites, milk, cilantro, salt, and pepper. Beat until fluffy.
2. In a 9-inch skillet over medium-low heat, add bacon strips and, once sizzling, turn heat to low. Flip bacon often until browned. Remove and place between paper towels to soak up excess oil.
3. Turn heat up to medium and add bell pepper and cumin. Cook until tender, about 3–4 minutes. Pour in egg mixture and gently push, lift, and fold eggs with spatula until set and cooked to desired doneness. Remove from heat and use the edge of spatula to cut egg mixture into chunks.
4. Warm tortillas in a small skillet about 1 minute each (or microwave 30 seconds). Divide egg mixture among tortillas, then add Cheddar, bacon, sour cream, and salsa. Serve.

Tomato and Leek Frittata

Onions are generally not allowed on the low-FODMAP diet, but you *can* use leek leaves, and they are delicious with eggs. Serve this frittata garnished with some extra goat cheese, tomato slices, and the green portions of sliced green onions.

Serves 2	
Per Serving	
Calories	258
Fat	18g
Protein	15g
Sodium	1,197mg
Fiber	2g
Carbohydrates	7g
Sugar	2g

3 teaspoons olive oil, divided

½ cup chopped leeks, dark green parts only

½ teaspoon sea salt, divided

½ teaspoon ground black pepper, divided

½ cup grape tomatoes

¼ cup capers, rinsed and drained

3 large egg whites

1 teaspoon herbes de Provence

1 teaspoon dried thyme

2 large egg yolks

2 ounces goat cheese, crumbled

1. Preheat oven to 350°F.
2. Heat 2 teaspoons oil in a 10-inch ovenproof nonstick skillet over medium heat. Add leeks, ¼ teaspoon salt, and ¼ teaspoon pepper. Cook 5 minutes. Stir in tomatoes and capers. Cover and cook 3 minutes. Transfer to a small bowl.
3. In a medium bowl, quickly beat egg whites with herbes de Provence, thyme, and remaining ¼ teaspoon salt and ¼ teaspoon pepper. Add egg yolks and continue whisking until mixture is fluffy.
4. Brush skillet with remaining 1 teaspoon oil. Add eggs, cooked tomato mixture, and goat cheese. Cook over medium heat 4 minutes.
5. Transfer to oven and bake 15–20 minutes or until eggs are set. (Check by cutting a small slit in center of frittata.) Serve.

Raspberry Lemon Oatmeal Bars

Raspberry and lemon are a flavor combination that is simply perfection! These bars are great to make ahead and have ready for a sweet and tasty breakfast on the go!

½ teaspoon turbinado sugar

1¼ cups unsweetened almond milk

½ teaspoon alcohol-free vanilla extract

1 large egg or Flax Egg (Chapter 2)

¼ cup pure maple syrup

3½ cups quick-cooking oats

2 tablespoons lemon juice

2 cups raspberries

Serves 12	
Per Serving	
Calories	127
Fat	2g
Protein	4g
Sodium	27mg
Fiber	4g
Carbohydrates	23g
Sugar	5g

1. Preheat oven to 350°F.
2. In a large bowl, whisk together sugar, almond milk, vanilla, egg, and syrup.
3. Add oats, lemon juice, and raspberries. Stir well to combine.
4. Pour into a 9" × 13" baking dish and bake 25 minutes. Cut into 12 bars and serve.

Cranberry Almond Granola

Throw this delicious, good-for-you granola on top of lactose-free yogurt, rice cereal, or quinoa flakes. You can store this granola in an airtight container for up to 3 weeks.

Serves 4

Per Serving

Calories	240
Fat	14g
Protein	3g
Sodium	2mg
Fiber	3g
Carbohydrates	26g
Sugar	10g

Cranberry Tip

For a softer texture, place dried cranberries in a small bowl with hot water and let stand for 20 minutes before draining and using. One tablespoon of dried cranberries is low in FODMAPs.

1 tablespoon chopped walnuts

1 tablespoon flaxseed

3 tablespoons canola oil

3 tablespoons pure maple syrup

¼ teaspoon alcohol-free vanilla extract

¼ teaspoon alcohol-free almond extract

1 cup rolled oats

1 tablespoon slivered almonds

½ teaspoon ground cinnamon

2 tablespoons no-sugar-added dried cranberries

1. In a small food chopper or blender, pulse walnuts until ground. Transfer to a large bowl. Next, pulse flaxseed until finely ground, and add to same large bowl.
2. In a medium bowl, stir together oil, syrup, and vanilla and almond extracts.
3. To the large bowl, add oats, almonds, and cinnamon and stir to combine with ground nuts. Pour oil mixture over top and stir well to combine.
4. Spread granola on a rimmed baking sheet, and bake 15 minutes. Stir occasionally to ensure granola turns a light-brown color all over.
5. After removing granola from oven, add cranberries and stir to combine. Serve.

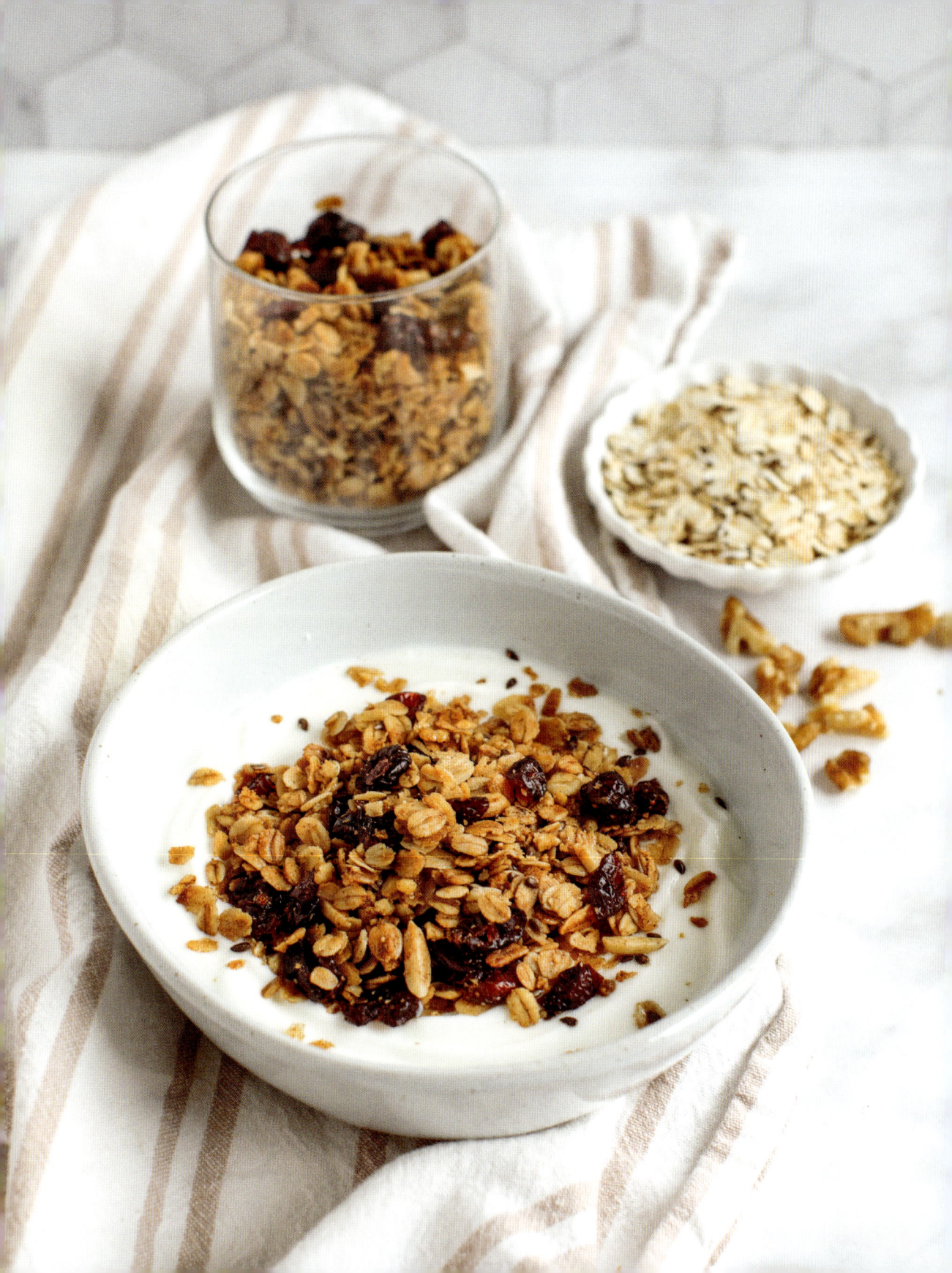

Overnight Peanut Butter Pumpkin Spice Oats

You will love digging into these hearty and delicious oats! They're perfect before a big day when you need some steady energy. These oats can be stored in the refrigerator for up to 3 days.

Serves 2

Per Serving

Calories 265
Fat 14g
Protein 8g
Sodium 27mg
Fiber 5g
Carbohydrates 28g
Sugar 10g

Overnight Oats Have So Many Possibilities!

Overnight oats are so easy to make, and there are several different variations you can try with foods low in FODMAPs. Just always be sure to use a 1:1 ratio for oats and almond milk (unless you like your oats runny). Be mindful of the appropriate recommended servings for the low-FODMAP diet to keep your overnight oats low in overall FODMAPs. One ¼-cup serving of oats is low-FODMAP.

½ cup rolled oats

¼ cup unsweetened almond milk

¼ cup pumpkin purée

½ teaspoon pumpkin pie spice

½ teaspoon alcohol-free vanilla extract

½ teaspoon ground cinnamon

1 tablespoon pure maple syrup

2 tablespoons peanut butter

2 tablespoons chopped walnuts

1. In a medium bowl, combine oats and almond milk and stir. Add pumpkin purée, pumpkin pie spice, vanilla, cinnamon, and syrup. Stir.
2. Spoon about ¼ of mixture into each of two small canning jars. Add 1 tablespoon peanut butter on top of oats in each jar. Then divide remaining oat mixture evenly between jars. Cover with lids. Refrigerate overnight.
3. In the morning, top with walnuts and serve.

Carrot Cake Overnight Oats with Walnuts

Who said you couldn't have cake in the morning? These overnight oats are a good-for-you breakfast that tastes like dessert—and they can be stored in the refrigerator for up to 3 days.

3 ounces lactose-free plain yogurt

¼ cup unsweetened almond milk

½ cup rolled oats

1 tablespoon chia seeds

¼ cup peeled and shredded carrots

2 tablespoons crushed pineapple

¼ teaspoon alcohol-free vanilla extract

½ tablespoon pure maple syrup

½ teaspoon ground cinnamon

1 tablespoon walnut halves

Serves 2	
Per Serving	
Calories	201
Fat	8g
Protein	6g
Sodium	54mg
Fiber	6g
Carbohydrates	28g
Sugar	8g

1. In a medium bowl, combine yogurt, almond milk, and oats, and stir. Add chia seeds, carrots, pineapple, vanilla, syrup, and cinnamon, and stir to combine. Place in two small canning jars and cover with lids. Refrigerate overnight.
2. In the morning, top with walnuts and serve.

Amaranth Breakfast

This recipe will make your home smell wonderful! It can be made in a rice cooker if you happen to have one. When serving, feel free to add a few drops of pure maple syrup and whatever berries you have on hand.

Serves 4	
Per Serving	
Calories	235
Fat	8g
Protein	7g
Sodium	1mg
Fiber	5g
Carbohydrates	35g
Sugar	1g

1 cup amaranth seeds

3 cups water

2 teaspoons ground cinnamon

1 teaspoon alcohol-free vanilla extract

¼ cup lightly chopped pecans

1. Heat a medium, heavy-bottomed saucepan over medium heat, and add amaranth. Toast, stirring occasionally, until fragrant, about 5 minutes.
2. Pour in water and bring to a boil. Lower heat to low and add cinnamon and vanilla. Cover and simmer 20 minutes, stirring occasionally.
3. While amaranth is simmering, place pecans under broiler 4 minutes to toast.
4. When amaranth has finished cooking, give it a good stir and remove from heat. Serve in bowls, topped with pecans.

CHAPTER 4

Appetizers and Snacks

Mini Baked Eggplant Pizza Bites

These baked pizza bites can be very addicting! And because they are baked, not fried, they're lower in fat than some pizza bites, which makes them a lighter snack option.

Serves 4

Per Serving

Calories 238
Fat 5g
Protein 7g
Sodium 612mg
Fiber 11g
Carbohydrates 42g
Sugar 10g

Gluten-Free Panko

A few brands of gluten-free, low-FODMAP panko (a type of bread crumbs) are available. Ian's is one. If you don't see them at your regular grocery store, look to a health food store, specialty grocer, or online retailer.

2 medium eggplants

½ teaspoon salt

1 large egg

¾ cup gluten-free panko

2 tablespoons dried oregano

2 teaspoons olive oil

½ cup Basic Marinara Sauce (Chapter 2)

¼ cup shredded mozzarella cheese

1. Preheat oven to 400°F.
2. Peel eggplants and cut off top and bottom ends, then cut into ½-inch round slices. Place in a colander and toss with salt. Let sit about 10 minutes. Rinse with water.
3. Whisk egg in a small bowl. Place panko in a medium, shallow bowl. Add oregano, stirring well to combine. Dredge each eggplant slice in egg, tap off any excess, and then dredge in bread crumbs. Place on a nonstick baking sheet.
4. Slowly drizzle oil to cover the top of each eggplant piece. Bake 12 minutes.
5. Remove eggplant from oven and spoon marinara sauce onto the center of each slice, leaving edges of eggplant uncovered. Sprinkle mozzarella on top. Bake 2–3 minutes or until cheese has melted. Serve.

Coconut Shrimp with Pineapple Sauce

No need to go out to a restaurant with questionable ingredients when you can make your own delicious coconut shrimp at home! These shrimp are great for parties and holidays, or to top a green salad any day of the year.

2½ cups chopped pineapple

2 tablespoons gluten-free fish sauce

1 tablespoon turbinado sugar

⅛ teaspoon wheat-free asafetida powder

1½ teaspoons Sweet Chili Garlic Sauce (Chapter 10)

1 tablespoon fresh lime juice

1 cup gluten-free panko

1½ cups shredded unsweetened coconut

½ teaspoon sea salt

2 large eggs

2 large egg whites

40 large, uncooked shrimp

Serves 8	
Per Serving	
Calories	159
Fat	6g
Protein	8g
Sodium	721mg
Fiber	3g
Carbohydrates	19g
Sugar	8g

1. Preheat oven to 425°F. Line a baking sheet with parchment paper.
2. In a blender or food processor, combine pineapple, fish sauce, sugar, asafetida, Sweet Chili Garlic Sauce, and lime juice. Process 45 seconds or until smooth. Place in a small serving bowl.
3. In a shallow bowl, combine panko, coconut, and salt. In a separate medium bowl, beat eggs and egg whites until light and airy.
4. Add ¼ of shrimp at a time to eggs, tossing to coat. Next, dredge shrimp in bread crumb mixture, then place on baking sheet. Repeat with all shrimp.
5. Bake 12 minutes. Halfway through cooking time, use tongs to lightly grab shrimp by tails to turn over. Serve with prepared pineapple sauce.

Indian-Spiced Mixed Nuts

These nuts make a great appetizer to hold over a hungry crowd, and they're equally good as a low-FODMAP snack to take along with you on your adventures.

How Many Nuts in a Low-FODMAP Serving?

On the low-FODMAP diet you can enjoy up to 18 assorted nuts, about 36 grams. Cashews and pistachios are high in FODMAPs and should be avoided. One low-FODMAP serving for almonds, hazelnuts, or Brazil nuts equals 10 nuts; for pecans, it's 10 halves. A low-FODMAP serving for chestnuts or macadamia nuts is 20 nuts, and for peanuts it's 32 nuts.

½ cup whole almonds

1 cup whole macadamia nuts

1 cup halved walnuts

1 cup halved pecans

1 teaspoon Himalayan sea salt

¼ teaspoon ground cumin

¾ teaspoon ground cinnamon

¼ teaspoon chili powder

¼ teaspoon ground turmeric

¼ teaspoon ground cardamom

½ teaspoon ground black pepper

½ cup light brown sugar

¼ cup water

1½ tablespoons unsalted butter

1. Preheat oven to 350°F. Line a baking sheet with aluminum foil and spray with cooking spray.
2. In a large bowl, combine almonds, macadamia nuts, walnuts, and pecans. Add salt, cumin, cinnamon, chili powder, turmeric, cardamom, and pepper. Toss to coat.
3. In a small saucepan over medium heat, heat sugar, water, and butter until butter is melted. Remove from heat. Carefully and slowly pour butter mixture over bowl of nuts, stirring to coat.
4. Transfer nuts to prepared baking sheet, spreading evenly in a single layer. Bake 10 minutes.
5. Remove and stir nuts, ensuring every nut gets coated and keeping all nuts in a single layer. Return to oven and bake 7 more minutes. Allow nuts to cool before serving.

Pão de Queijo (Cheese Bread)

Pão de Queijo is a small, cheesy roll that's a popular snack and breakfast food in Brazil. These cheesy delights are also great served alongside your favorite stew or roast.

1 cup lactose-free milk

½ cup coconut oil

1 teaspoon sea salt

2 cups tapioca starch

2 large eggs, whisked

1½ cups grated Parmesan cheese

Olive oil for handling dough

Makes 2 dozen rolls

**Per Serving
(Serving size: 2 rolls)**

Calories 229
Fat 13g
Protein 5g
Sodium 377mg
Fiber 0g
Carbohydrates 21g
Sugar 1g

1. Preheat oven to 450°F. Line two baking sheets with parchment paper.
2. In a medium saucepan over medium heat, combine milk, oil, and salt. Whisking occasionally, bring to a slow boil. Once you see large bubbles, remove pan from heat.
3. Add starch to saucepan and stir until well combined. Dough should have a gelatinous texture.
4. Transfer dough to the bowl of a stand mixer. With a paddle attachment, beat dough at medium speed 5–7 minutes or until smooth.
5. Still at medium speed, slowly add eggs. Use a spatula to scrape down any dough stuck to sides of bowl.
6. Add Parmesan and continue to beat on medium speed until fully incorporated. Dough should be very sticky, stretchy, and soft.
7. Using a tablespoon measure or ice cream scoop, make rounded balls of dough and place them on baking sheets 1 to 2 inches apart. Dip your fingers in a bowl of olive oil to keep dough from sticking to your hands.
8. Place in oven, and immediately turn heat down to 350°F. Bake 25–30 minutes. Remove once outsides are dry and flecked with orange. Serve.

Herbes de Provence Almonds

These savory roasted almonds are easy to make and are a healthy low-FODMAP snack you can eat on the go.

What Is a Suitable Serving of Almonds?

When enjoying Herbes de Provence Almonds or other almond recipes in this book, stick to a low-FODMAP serving of 10 almonds. Larger serving sizes should be avoided, as almonds contain high amounts of galacto-oligosaccharides (GOS).

1½ tablespoons unsalted butter, melted

1½ teaspoons herbes de Provence, crushed

½ teaspoon sea salt

⅛ teaspoon paprika

1 cup raw almonds

1. Preheat oven to 350°F.
2. In a medium bowl, combine butter, herbes de Provence, salt, and paprika. Add almonds and toss to coat.
3. Scatter almonds evenly on a rimmed baking sheet.
4. Bake 10–12 minutes, stirring halfway through the cooking time.
5. When toasted and fragrant, remove from oven and serve warm.

Baked Camembert and Rosemary

Thankfully, on the low-FODMAP diet you can enjoy such heavenly things as Camembert cheese! Stick to about 1.4 ounces for a low-FODMAP serving.

1 (8-ounce) box Camembert cheese

5 sprigs rosemary

2 tablespoons dry white wine

1 tablespoon pure maple syrup

½ teaspoon ground black pepper

18 (about ½-ounce) slices gluten-free baguette

2 tablespoons garlic-infused olive oil, divided

1 teaspoon coarse sea salt

Serves 7	
Per Serving	
Calories	218
Fat	14g
Protein	8g
Sodium	639mg
Fiber	1g
Carbohydrates	15g
Sugar	2g

1. Remove cheese from refrigerator 1 hour before cooking and bring to room temperature.
2. Preheat oven to 315°F. Take cheese out of box and unwrap.
3. Remove any waxed paper from box. Nest box base inside of lid, and return cheese to box. Place on a rimmed baking sheet. Make five slits in top of cheese, and place rosemary inside slits. Pour wine and maple syrup into slits and on top of cheese. Sprinkle on pepper.
4. Bake 20 minutes. After 12 minutes have passed, add baguette slices to baking sheet, drizzle bread with 1 tablespoon oil, and sprinkle with salt.
5. Remove baking sheet from oven and allow to cool. Drizzle cheese with remaining 1 tablespoon oil. Serve with baguette slices.

Kale Chips

There's no need to buy expensive kale chips from the store when you can make your own earthy and delicious version at home. Kale has a long list of possible health benefits, so munch away!

Serves 4	
Per Serving	
Calories	67
Fat	7g
Protein	1g
Sodium	82mg
Fiber	1g
Carbohydrates	1g
Sugar	0g

1 large bunch curly kale, stems removed, torn into bite-sized pieces

2 tablespoons olive oil

¼ teaspoon ground turmeric

½ teaspoon curry powder

½ teaspoon chili powder

½ teaspoon ground cumin

⅛ teaspoon coarse salt

1. Preheat oven to 350°F. Line two baking sheets with parchment paper.
2. Put kale in a large bowl and drizzle with oil. Add turmeric, curry powder, chili powder, and cumin. Massage kale until evenly coated. Add more oil if all pieces are still not evenly coated.
3. Spread kale pieces in a single layer on baking sheets and sprinkle with salt.
4. Bake 16 minutes, rotating pans after 8 minutes. Bake until crispy. Serve immediately.

Chocolate Chip Energy Bites

When you need a little bit of energy on an active day, try these delicious, chocolaty, and nutty energy bites. These snacks can be stored in a freezer bag in the freezer for up to 2 weeks.

½ cup oat bran

½ cup almond butter

⅓ cup pure maple syrup

1½ cups quick-cooking oats

¼ cup pumpkin seeds

¼ cup dark chocolate chips

¼ cup no-sugar-added dried cranberries

¼ cup ground walnuts

1. Preheat oven to 375°F.
2. Add oat bran to a baking sheet and toast 5–7 minutes or until lightly brown.
3. Using a handheld or stand mixer, mix together almond butter and syrup on low speed until well combined.
4. Continuing to mix, gradually add oats until combined, and then add pumpkin seeds, chocolate chips, cranberries, and walnuts. Mix until well combined.
5. Line a second baking sheet with parchment paper.
6. Gently roll oat mixture into 24 even balls.
7. Roll balls in toasted oat bran and place on baking sheet. Refrigerate 2 hours to set, or consume immediately.

Coconut Cinnamon Popcorn

When made the right way, popcorn can be very healthy. This recipe has 3 grams of fiber per serving, which is great for the digestion! Try this recipe on your next movie night.

Serves 2	
Per Serving	
Calories	183
Fat	13g
Protein	2g
Sodium	1mg
Fiber	3g
Carbohydrates	14g
Sugar	0g

Choosing the Right Popcorn

When buying microwavable popcorn, choose a brand that contains as few ingredients as possible beyond popcorn kernels. Stay away from brands that use added salt, diacetyl (a synthetic butter flavoring), other artificial flavorings, TBHQ (tertiary butylhydroquinone, a fat preservative), and propyl gallate (an artificial food additive).

2 tablespoons coconut oil

½ tablespoon ground cinnamon

4 cups freshly popped popcorn

1. Add coconut oil and cinnamon to a microwave-safe measuring cup. Microwave 30 seconds or until coconut oil has melted. Stir to combine.
2. Pour coconut and cinnamon mixture over popcorn, and shake to combine. (If using microwavable popcorn, you can do this right in the bag.) Serve.

Fiesta Nachos

Planning a fun night in? Try these fun nachos with all the low-FODMAP fixings.

½ pound lean ground beef

¼ teaspoon chili powder

¼ teaspoon dried oregano

¼ teaspoon paprika

¼ teaspoon ground cumin

⅛ teaspoon salt

⅛ teaspoon ground black pepper

1 tablespoon safflower oil

35 tortilla chips

½ cup Fiesta Salsa (Chapter 10)

¼ cup sliced black olives

1½ cups shredded Cheddar cheese

2 green onions, chopped, green parts only

½ cup lactose-free sour cream

Serves 4	
Per Serving	
Calories	483
Fat	30g
Protein	25g
Sodium	721mg
Fiber	2g
Carbohydrates	23g
Sugar	4g

1. Preheat oven to 350°F. Spray a 9" × 13" baking dish with cooking spray.
2. In a medium bowl, add beef, chili powder, oregano, paprika, cumin, salt, and pepper and mix together with hands.
3. Set a large skillet over medium-high heat and add beef mixture and oil. Cook 5 minutes, chopping up beef with a spatula into bite-sized pieces as you cook. Set aside.
4. Line baking dish with tortilla chips. Sprinkle on beef, salsa, olives, cheese, and green onions.
5. Bake 10 minutes or until cheese is melted. Top with sour cream. Serve immediately.

Roasted Pumpkin Seeds

When cooking with pumpkin or carving a jack-o'-lantern in the fall, don't throw away the seeds—use them for roasting! They're so easy to cook, and they make a delicious low-FODMAP snack!

Makes 1 cup	
Per Serving	
(Serving size: ½ cup)	
Calories	420
Fat	36g
Protein	20g
Sodium	585mg
Fiber	4g
Carbohydrates	7g
Sugar	1g

1 cup pumpkin seeds, rinsed and dried

1 tablespoon olive oil

½ teaspoon salt

1. Preheat oven to 300°F. Line a rimmed baking sheet with parchment paper.
2. In a medium bowl, toss together all ingredients. Spread mixture in a single layer on baking sheet.
3. Bake 50–60 minutes, stirring every 15 minutes until seeds are crisp. Let cool completely before serving. Store in a sealed container at room temperature.

Dark Chocolate–Covered Pretzels

Who doesn't love chocolate-covered pretzels? It is a classic taste combination. Have these on hand when you need a sweet and salty low-FODMAP fix.

Makes 12 pretzels	
Per Serving	
(Serving size: 4 pretzels)	
Calories	164
Fat	11g
Protein	1g
Sodium	76mg
Fiber	1g
Carbohydrates	15g
Sugar	8g

3 ounces dark chocolate chips

1 tablespoon vegetable shortening

12 gluten-free mini pretzels

1. Melt chocolate and shortening over a double boiler. Stir until smooth and combined.
2. Remove from heat. Dip each pretzel in chocolate, allowing excess to drip off.
3. Place on a baking sheet lined with waxed paper and chill in refrigerator until firm. Serve.

CHAPTER 5

Poultry, Pork, and Beef

Pork and Fennel Meatballs

These meatballs can be described as earthy and definitely tasty. Serve either as appetizers or as a full meal with gluten-free pasta and the Basic Marinara Sauce from Chapter 2 with a sprinkle of chopped parsley.

Makes 24 meatballs	
Per Serving **(Serving size: 3 meatballs)**	
Calories	122
Fat	5g
Protein	13g
Sodium	151mg
Fiber	1g
Carbohydrates	4g
Sugar	0g

1 pound lean ground pork

2 tablespoons roughly chopped flat-leaf parsley

3 tablespoons gluten-free panko

1 large egg

1/8 teaspoon wheat-free asafetida powder

1/4 teaspoon salt

1/2 teaspoon ground black pepper

1 1/2 tablespoons olive oil

2 teaspoons fennel seeds

1. In a large mixing bowl, combine pork, parsley, panko, egg, asafetida, salt, and pepper. Stir to combine, or mix well with hands. Shape into 1-inch meatballs.
2. In a medium skillet, heat oil over medium heat and toast fennel seeds until fragrant, about 4 minutes. Add meatballs to pan.
3. Brown meatballs on all sides, cooking about 4–5 minutes per side, 20 minutes total, until cooked through and no longer pink inside. Serve.

Roast Beef Tenderloin with Parmesan Crust

If you like roast beef, you'll love it even more when it's coated with a lovely Parmesan crust.

1 (4-pound) center-cut beef tenderloin, fat and silver skin trimmed

¼ teaspoon kosher salt

5 teaspoons ground black pepper, divided

⅔ cup gluten-free fine bread crumbs

¾ cup finely grated Parmesan cheese

⅔ cup Basic Mayonnaise (Chapter 2)

1 tablespoon Dijon mustard

1 tablespoon finely grated lemon zest

1 tablespoon gluten-free Worcestershire sauce

Serves 8	
Per Serving	
Calories	518
Fat	25g
Protein	54g
Sodium	545mg
Fiber	1g
Carbohydrates	14g
Sugar	1g

Tips on Buying Beef Tenderloin

If you want to purchase a roast completely trimmed and don't mind paying extra, just ask your butcher to prepare it "side muscle off and skinned."

1. Season tenderloin lightly with salt and 1 teaspoon pepper. Wrap in plastic wrap and refrigerate overnight.
2. The next day, uncover tenderloin and let stand at room temperature up to, but not exceeding, 2 hours.
3. Preheat oven to 400°F.
4. Set a rack inside a rimmed baking sheet. Spray rack with nonstick cooking spray. Transfer tenderloin to rack.
5. In a food processor, pulse remaining 4 teaspoons pepper and remaining ingredients until well blended. Using your hands, pack Parmesan mixture around tenderloin.
6. Roast until crust is golden brown, about 30–40 minutes for medium-rare. An instant-read thermometer inserted into the thickest part of the tenderloin should register 120°F–125°F.
7. Transfer to a carving board and cover loosely with foil. Let rest 10 minutes. Cut into ½-inch-thick slices, being careful to keep the delicate crust in place. Serve.

Stuffed Peppers with Ground Turkey

Enjoy these stuffed peppers as a side dish or main dish. Alternatively, try ground chicken or a different low-FODMAP cheese.

Serves 3

Per Serving

Calories 840
Fat 51g
Protein 51g
Sodium 461mg
Fiber 6g
Carbohydrates 39g
Sugar 9g

How to Roast Corn in the Oven

For oven-roasted corn, first preheat your oven to 450°F. Remove the husks and silk threads from 2 ears of corn. Rub the corn cobs with 1 tablespoon of butter, and wrap them in foil. Place them on a rimmed baking sheet, and roast for 20–25 minutes.

1 tablespoon olive oil

1 pound ground turkey

1 tablespoon garlic-infused olive oil, divided

1 cup roasted corn kernels

2 medium Roma tomatoes, chopped

2 tablespoons pine nuts

1 cup cooked brown rice

½ tablespoon chili powder

½ teaspoon ground cumin

1 teaspoon smoked paprika

3 tablespoons chopped cilantro

3 large bell peppers (orange, yellow, and green), halved and seeded

2 tablespoons coconut oil

6 ounces goat cheese

3 tablespoons Fiesta Salsa (Chapter 10)

1. Preheat oven to 375°F.
2. In a large skillet over medium-high heat, warm olive oil. Add turkey and cook, breaking meat apart with a spatula, 5–7 minutes, until browned.
3. Add ½ tablespoon garlic-infused oil to skillet, along with corn, tomatoes, and pine nuts. Stir and heat through.
4. Add rice and stir to combine. Stir in remaining ½ tablespoon garlic-infused oil, chili powder, cumin, paprika, and cilantro. Remove from heat.
5. Stuff halved peppers with brown rice mixture and brush outsides of peppers with coconut oil. Place peppers in an 8" × 8" shallow baking dish.
6. Top each pepper with an ounce of goat cheese. Loosely cover dish with foil.
7. Bake 30–40 minutes until peppers are tender. Garnish with salsa and serve.

Pork Chops with Carrots and Toasted Buckwheat

The sweetness of the carrots combined with the salt from the pork along with the earthy buckwheat makes this an all-around beautiful and pleasing dish. Filling and hearty dishes like this will satisfy your comfort-food cravings while you take care of your gut health!

1½ pounds carrots, peeled, halved lengthwise, and cut into 2-inch pieces

⅛ teaspoon wheat-free asafetida powder

4 teaspoons fresh lemon juice

¼ cup dill sprigs

2 tablespoons olive oil

½ teaspoon kosher salt, divided

1 medium orange, cut in half

¾ cup buckwheat groats

1 tablespoon safflower oil

2 (1-inch-thick) bone-in pork shoulder chops (about 8–10 ounces each)

2 tablespoons unsalted butter, divided

Serves 4

Per Serving

Calories	540
Fat	27g
Protein	31g
Sodium	431mg
Fiber	8g
Carbohydrates	41g
Sugar	9g

1. Preheat oven to 450°F.
2. In a medium bowl, place carrots, asafetida, lemon juice, dill, and olive oil. Toss well to coat. Place on a rimmed baking sheet and season with ¼ teaspoon salt. Roast carrots until tender and browned, tossing once, about 20 minutes.
3. Remove carrots from oven. Squeeze juice from ½ orange over carrots. Set aside.
4. Meanwhile, in a large saucepan of salted boiling water, cook buckwheat until tender, 10–15 minutes. Drain and rinse well under cold water, rinsing away any pinkish-red film (this is mucilage, a natural part of the buckwheat). Spread out on a baking sheet and allow to dry.
5. In a 10-inch heavy or cast iron skillet, heat safflower oil over high heat. Season pork with remaining ¼ teaspoon salt, and cook until browned and slightly pink in the center, about 5–6 minutes per side. Transfer to a cutting board.
6. Add buckwheat and 1 tablespoon butter to the same skillet. Cook 5 minutes, stirring frequently. Remove from heat. Divide buckwheat among four plates.
7. Add remaining 1 tablespoon butter to skillet, and squeeze in juice from remaining orange half. Heat until butter has melted.
8. Thinly slice pork. Top buckwheat with pork slices and carrots. Drizzle with orange-butter mixture and serve.

Lemon Thyme Chicken

Thyme is one of many beautiful herbs that you can use on the low-FODMAP diet, and it dresses chicken perfectly. Serve this dish with Lemon Kale Salad (Chapter 9).

Serves 4	
Per Serving	
Calories	550
Fat	30g
Protein	57g
Sodium	366mg
Fiber	0g
Carbohydrates	2g
Sugar	1g

4 skin-on chicken thighs and 4 drumsticks (about 2½ pounds total)

3 medium lemons

1 tablespoon unsalted butter, melted

¼ teaspoon sea salt

½ teaspoon ground black pepper

2 tablespoons thyme leaves

6 basil leaves, torn

1. Preheat oven to 375°F.
2. Add chicken to a large bowl. Grate zest of 1 lemon into bowl. Slice all 3 lemons in half, and juice into bowl.
3. Add butter, salt, pepper, and thyme, and toss well with your hands. Place chicken in a 9" × 13" baking dish.
4. Bake 35–40 minutes, basting every 10 minutes. Skin should get crispy, and meat should be cooked through.
5. Garnish with basil leaves and serve.

Spinach and Feta–Stuffed Chicken Breast

This recipe is relatively easy to make and only needs a few ingredients, including low-FODMAP ingredients that you may have on hand.

1 tablespoon garlic-infused olive oil

7 cups whole spinach leaves

½ cup crumbled feta cheese

2 (6-ounce) boneless, skinless chicken breasts, pounded to a ¼-inch thickness

1 large egg, lightly beaten

1 cup gluten-free bread crumbs

Serves 2	
Per Serving	
Calories	530
Fat	20g
Protein	50g
Sodium	773mg
Fiber	5g
Carbohydrates	39g
Sugar	3g

1. Preheat oven to 350°F.
2. Heat oil in a medium skillet over low heat. Add spinach, and cook until soft, 2–3 minutes. Add feta, stir a few times, and remove from heat.
3. Lay half of spinach mixture on top of each chicken breast. Wrap meat around mixture, and secure with toothpicks.
4. Place egg in a shallow bowl. Place bread crumbs in a separate shallow bowl. Roll each breast in egg, tap off any excess, then roll in bread crumbs until well coated.
5. Place in an 8" × 8" casserole dish. Bake 30 minutes, and serve warm.

Chicken Piccata

This is a delicious, quick, and flourless chicken piccata recipe. It's also soy-free and nut-free. If your capers are salt-packed, rinse them before using, and if they're brine-packed, drain them.

Serves 4	
Per Serving	
Calories	294
Fat	14g
Protein	37g
Sodium	1,046mg
Fiber	1g
Carbohydrates	2g
Sugar	1g

Make It a Seafood Piccata

Fish is another nice option to use in this recipe instead of chicken. Choose a light fish, such as flounder, red snapper, tilapia, or rainbow trout. Cook the fish until it easily flakes apart with a fork.

4 (6-ounce, ½– ¾-inch-thick) boneless, skinless chicken breasts

2 teaspoons sea salt

4 tablespoons unsalted butter, divided

2 tablespoons dry white wine

¼ cup capers

½ cup halved cherry tomatoes

2 teaspoons finely chopped flat-leaf parsley

2 large lemons, halved

1. Sprinkle all sides of chicken breasts with salt.
2. In a 10-inch skillet over medium-high heat, melt 2 tablespoons butter. Add chicken, and cook until opaque halfway through, 4–5 minutes.
3. Add wine and 1 more tablespoon butter to skillet. As soon as butter is melted, flip chicken and finish cooking through, 3–4 minutes. Transfer chicken to a serving platter.
4. Add capers to hot skillet, and let sizzle 30 seconds. Add tomatoes, parsley, and remaining 1 tablespoon butter. Squeeze juice from lemons into skillet, and stir everything to combine.
5. Cook another 30 seconds, then drizzle mixture over chicken. Serve immediately.

Easy Sheet Pan Chicken

This dish makes for a comforting home-cooked meal that's easy to assemble, ready in less than 45 minutes, and low-FODMAP to boot.

3 tablespoons whole-grain mustard

2 teaspoons dried oregano

1 teaspoon dried thyme

1 tablespoon unsalted butter, softened

2 teaspoons Dijon mustard

3 pounds bone-in chicken thighs and drumsticks, patted dry

½ teaspoon salt

1 teaspoon ground black pepper

⅔ cup gluten-free bread crumbs

4 medium carrots, peeled and halved lengthwise

1 tablespoon garlic-infused olive oil

Serves 4	
Per Serving	
Calories	754
Fat	43g
Protein	63g
Sodium	1,241mg
Fiber	4g
Carbohydrates	32g
Sugar	4g

1. Heat oven to 425°F. Line a baking sheet with parchment paper.
2. In a small bowl, combine whole-grain mustard, oregano, thyme, butter, and Dijon mustard.
3. Season chicken with salt and pepper. Rub mustard-butter mixture all over chicken.
4. Place bread crumbs in a wide bowl, dredge chicken to coat evenly, and place on baking sheet.
5. Place carrots (cut sides down) alongside chicken, and drizzle with oil.
6. Bake until chicken is golden and no longer pink inside, 35–40 minutes. Serve.

Blueberry-Glazed Chicken

While blueberries and chicken may seem like an odd flavor combination at first, this dish will make you a believer in no time. Sweet blueberry jam and maple syrup mixed with tart vinegar and lemon juice make this dish sing. Enjoy this delectable chicken dish with mashed potatoes or jasmine rice.

Serves 4

Per Serving

Calories 292
Fat 16g
Protein 25g
Sodium 398mg
Fiber 1g
Carbohydrates 11g
Sugar 8g

2 tablespoons balsamic vinegar

2 tablespoons olive oil

2 tablespoons lemon juice

2 teaspoons Dijon mustard

⅓ cup Blueberry Chia Seed Jam (Chapter 10)

1 tablespoon pure maple syrup

½ teaspoon salt

2 tablespoons coconut oil

4 (4-ounce) boneless, skinless chicken breasts

1. In a medium bowl, combine vinegar, oil, lemon juice, mustard, jam, syrup, and salt. Set aside.
2. Heat coconut oil in a large skillet over medium heat. Add chicken breasts, and brown on both sides.
3. Reduce heat to low, and add blueberry sauce. Cover and simmer until cooked through, about 20 minutes.
4. Spoon sauce over chicken to serve.

Pumpkin Maple-Roasted Chicken

Once in the oven, this simple roast chicken with pumpkin, maple syrup, cinnamon, and thyme will cast a fragrant spell over your kitchen. After carving, be sure to drizzle each serving with Pumpkin Maple Glaze (Chapter 10).

1½ tablespoons unsalted butter

1 tablespoon canned pumpkin

1 tablespoon pure maple syrup

1 teaspoon ground cinnamon

1 teaspoon dried thyme

½ teaspoon sea salt

¼ teaspoon ground black pepper

1 (4-pound) whole chicken

Serves 4	
Per Serving	
Calories	497
Fat	27g
Protein	50g
Sodium	348mg
Fiber	1g
Carbohydrates	4g
Sugar	3g

1. Preheat oven to 375°F.
2. In a small saucepan over medium-low heat, melt butter. Add pumpkin, syrup, cinnamon, thyme, salt, and pepper, and stir until combined. Refrigerate 10 minutes.
3. Cut small slits under skin on both sides of chicken breast and under legs. Once the pumpkin mixture is cool, generously rub it under skin and all over top of skin. Spray rack of a roasting pan with nonstick cooking spray. Place chicken, breast side up, on the rack. Roast 50–60 minutes or until a meat thermometer registers 165°F at thickest part of thigh.
4. Tent with foil and let rest 5 minutes before carving.

Canned Pumpkin

Be cautious when purchasing canned pumpkin! A very similar-looking canned product, known as pumpkin pie filling, contains ingredients that may not be appropriate for a low-FODMAP diet. Pure canned pumpkin should have just one ingredient—pumpkin—and so can be enjoyed without worry.

Polenta-Crusted Chicken

You don't need a heavy batter coating that could cause your symptoms to flare!
Low-FODMAP polenta makes a deliciously crunchy and very fulfilling crust for your
chicken! Serve this dish with spinach, green beans, or a generous salad.

Serves 2

Per Serving

Calories	525
Fat	23g
Protein	43g
Sodium	680mg
Fiber	1g
Carbohydrates	33g
Sugar	0g

1 large egg

½ teaspoon salt, divided

½ teaspoon ground black pepper, divided

¼ cup gluten-free all-purpose flour

¼ cup quick-cooking polenta

1 teaspoon dried oregano

1 teaspoon dried thyme

¾ pound boneless, skinless chicken breasts

¼ cup safflower oil

¼ cup olive oil

1. In a shallow bowl, beat egg with ¼ teaspoon each salt and pepper. In another shallow bowl, whisk together flour, polenta, oregano, thyme, and remaining ¼ teaspoon each salt and pepper.
2. Dip chicken in egg, tapping off any excess, then dredge in polenta mixture.
3. Heat safflower oil and olive oil in a 6-inch nonstick skillet over medium heat.
4. Cook chicken in batches until golden brown, 4–6 minutes on one side and 2 minutes on other side. Serve.

Barbecue Pork Macaroni and Cheese

This sweet and savory blend of flavors is a real crowd-pleaser. Remove the meats and Parmesan cheese, substitute a low-FODMAP vegetable stock (Chapter 2) for the chicken stock, and this recipe makes a wonderful vegetarian main dish.

1 pound gluten-free macaroni, cooked al dente and drained

1½ cups peeled and cubed butternut squash

1 teaspoon extra-virgin olive oil

1 teaspoon sea salt, divided

½ teaspoon ground black pepper, divided

¼ teaspoon ground nutmeg

¼ teaspoon ground ginger

½ pound boneless pork loin, cut into ½-inch cubes

¼ cup Sweet Barbecue Sauce (Chapter 2)

¾ cup Easy Onion- and Garlic-Free Chicken Stock (Chapter 2)

¾ cup coconut milk

1½ cups shredded Cheddar cheese, divided

1 cup (loosely packed) thinly sliced kale

2 slices bacon, cooked, cooled, and crumbled

½ cup grated Parmesan cheese

Serves 8	
Per Serving	
Calories	296
Fat	17g
Protein	17g
Sodium	565mg
Fiber	1g
Carbohydrates	27g
Sugar	2g

1. Place cooked macaroni in a 9" × 13" baking dish, and set aside.
2. Heat oven to 375°F. On a parchment paper–lined baking sheet, toss squash with oil. Sprinkle with ½ teaspoon salt, ¼ teaspoon pepper, nutmeg, and ginger. Bake 25 minutes. Remove from oven and set aside to cool.
3. In a medium skillet over medium heat, brown pork on all sides. Add barbecue sauce, and toss to coat. Simmer, uncovered, 1–2 minutes. Remove from heat, and set aside to cool.
4. Transfer cooled squash to the bowl of a food processor. Add stock, coconut milk, and remaining ½ teaspoon salt and ¼ teaspoon pepper, and process to combine. Add 1 cup Cheddar and pulse until combined.
5. Pour squash mixture over macaroni in baking dish, and stir to combine.
6. Tuck kale here and there among the noodles. Dot top of casserole evenly with barbecue pork cubes and bacon.
7. Sprinkle top of casserole evenly with Parmesan and remaining ½ cup Cheddar. Bake 20 minutes or until cheese is melted and bubbling. Let sit 5 minutes, then serve.

Turkey and Kale Pasta

This one-pot, one-pan meal is quick and easy to make and effortless to customize—discover a new tasty variation by adding other low-FODMAP ingredients.

Serves 4

Per Serving

Calories	398
Fat	20g
Protein	32g
Sodium	471mg
Fiber	3g
Carbohydrates	29g
Sugar	4g

½ pound gluten-free pasta

2 cups chopped kale (ribs and stems removed)

2 tablespoons extra-virgin olive oil, divided

1⁄16 teaspoon salt

1 large carrot, peeled and thinly sliced

½ medium stalk celery, thinly sliced

1 tablespoon dried oregano

½ teaspoon ground black pepper

1 pound lean ground turkey

½ cup Easy Onion- and Garlic-Free Chicken Stock (Chapter 2)

1 (13.5-ounce) can diced tomatoes

3 tablespoons chopped flat-leaf parsley

6 black olives, sliced

¾ cup grated mozzarella cheese

1. Cook pasta according to package directions.
2. Meanwhile, add kale to a small bowl with 1 tablespoon oil and salt. Massage until leaves are soft. Set aside.
3. Heat a large saucepan with remaining 1 tablespoon oil over medium-high heat. Add carrots, celery, oregano, and pepper, and sauté until carrots are tender, about 8–10 minutes.
4. Add turkey, and break up into bite-sized pieces with spatula. Cook until browned, about 5–7 minutes. Add stock, tomatoes, and parsley, and reduce heat to low. Cook, covered, 5 minutes.
5. Once pasta is cooked and drained, add to saucepan. Stir in kale, olives, and mozzarella, and toss to combine. Remove from heat. Cover and let rest 2 minutes, then serve.

Crispy Baked Chicken with Gravy

When you're in the mood for a cozy dish, this chicken and rice recipe will hit the spot. Warm, filling, and covered in luxurious gravy, this chicken dish lets you know you aren't missing out on anything!

2 cups brown rice

4 cups plus 2 tablespoons water, divided

2½ pounds boneless, skinless chicken breasts

1 cup gluten-free panko

4 tablespoons olive oil, divided

2 tablespoons minced flat-leaf parsley

¼ cup Dijon mustard

¼ teaspoon salt, divided

½ teaspoon ground black pepper, divided

6 tablespoons unsalted butter

½ cup plus 6 tablespoons gluten-free all-purpose flour

1 cup lactose-free milk

1 cup Easy Onion- and Garlic-Free Chicken Stock (Chapter 2)

¼ teaspoon dried thyme

Serves 4	
Per Serving	
Calories	1,251
Fat	41g
Protein	77g
Sodium	1,046mg
Fiber	7g
Carbohydrates	134g
Sugar	3g

1. Place rice and 4 cups water in a medium saucepan. Bring to a boil, reduce heat to low, and cover. Allow to simmer 20 minutes until rice is tender. Remove from heat, stir, and keep covered. Set aside.

2. Preheat oven to 400°F. Line a rimmed baking sheet with aluminum foil. Place a rack in pan, and spray rack with nonstick cooking spray.

3. Using a meat tenderizer, pound each chicken breast to a ¼-inch thickness. Set aside.

4. In a shallow dish, combine panko, 2 tablespoons oil, and parsley. In a separate shallow dish, combine mustard, remaining 2 tablespoons water, ⅛ teaspoon salt, ¼ teaspoon pepper, and remaining 2 tablespoons oil.

5. Coat each chicken breast with mustard mixture; dredge each in bread crumb mixture. Place on prepared rack in pan.

6. Bake 25–30 minutes or until chicken is golden brown.

7. About 15–20 minutes into baking chicken, begin preparing gravy: Over medium heat, melt butter in a medium saucepan, and whisk in flour to make a roux. Whisk constantly until mixture bubbles and flour turns light brown in color. Gradually whisk in milk, stock, and thyme, and continue to stir. Add remaining ⅛ teaspoon salt and ¼ teaspoon pepper. Mixture should thicken after about 5 minutes.

8. Divide rice onto four plates. Place chicken breasts on rice, and spoon gravy on top. Serve immediately.

CHAPTER 6

Fish and Shellfish

Seafood Risotto

Creamy risotto serves as the base for plump clams, shrimp, and scallops. Luscious dishes like this one not only will keep you feeling satisfied on your low-FODMAP diet but may become some of your new favorite things to eat! This dish is best paired with something light, such as a basic green salad.

Serves 6	
Per Serving	
Calories	440
Fat	18g
Protein	20g
Sodium	911mg
Fiber	1g
Carbohydrates	44g
Sugar	0g

2½ cups water

2 (8-ounce) bottles clam juice

6 tablespoons olive oil, divided

1½ cups Arborio rice

½ cup dry white wine

¾ pound large, uncooked shrimp, peeled, deveined, and coarsely chopped

¾ pound bay scallops

⅛ teaspoon wheat-free asafetida powder

1 tablespoon salted butter

½ cup grated Parmesan cheese

2 tablespoons finely chopped flat-leaf parsley

1. Combine water and clam juice in a medium saucepan. Bring to a simmer and keep warm over low heat.
2. In a heavy, large saucepan over medium heat, warm 3 tablespoons oil. Add rice and sauté 2 minutes.
3. Add wine, and stir until liquid is absorbed, about 2 minutes. Add 1 cup clam juice mixture to rice. Simmer until liquid is absorbed, stirring often. Continue adding clam juice mixture ½ cup at a time, stirring often and simmering until liquid is absorbed before each addition. Simmer until rice is tender but still slightly firm in center and mixture is creamy, about 25 minutes.
4. Heat remaining 3 tablespoons oil in a heavy, large skillet over medium-high heat. Add shrimp, scallops, and asafetida. Sauté until centers of shrimp and scallops are opaque, about 6 minutes.
5. Add seafood to rice. Stir, add butter, and cook 4 minutes longer. Remove from heat, and stir in Parmesan. Transfer to serving bowl.
6. Garnish with parsley and serve.

Shrimp and Cheese Casserole

The creaminess of mozzarella and the sharp, pleasant tang of feta fill this dish with warm, cheesy goodness. This Greek-inspired low-FODMAP dish is delicious paired with mashed potatoes and a green salad.

3 tablespoons unsalted butter

⅛ teaspoon salt

⅛ teaspoon ground black pepper

⅛ teaspoon wheat-free asafetida powder

¼ cup dry white wine

10 ounces fresh spinach, chopped

1 (14.5-ounce) can diced tomatoes, drained

10 ounces medium shrimp, peeled and deveined

2 tablespoons olive oil

¼ pound crumbled feta cheese

¼ pound shredded mozzarella cheese

Serves 4	
Per Serving	
Calories	394
Fat	26g
Protein	23g
Sodium	1,170mg
Fiber	3g
Carbohydrates	12g
Sugar	5g

1. Preheat oven to 350°F. Grease a 9" × 13" casserole dish.
2. In a large skillet, melt butter over medium-high heat. Add salt, pepper, and asafetida, and stir. Add wine and spinach, and cook 2–3 minutes until spinach wilts.
3. Put spinach mixture into prepared casserole dish, and layer in tomatoes. Place shrimp on top, and drizzle with oil. Sprinkle with feta and mozzarella.
4. Bake 25 minutes or until cheese is bubbly and slightly brown. Serve.

Grilled Swordfish with Pineapple Salsa

This fish dish is perfect for a summer day when you don't want to turn your oven on. Get your grill fired up and enjoy this recipe with a crisp green salad.

Serves 4

Per Serving

Calories	269
Fat	12g
Protein	20g
Sodium	201mg
Fiber	2g
Carbohydrates	18g
Sugar	13g

2 tablespoons finely chopped cilantro

2 medium limes, juiced and zested

1 medium orange, juiced and zested

½ medium pineapple, cut into small chunks

¼ teaspoon kosher salt

½ teaspoon ground black pepper

4 (3.5-ounce, 1-inch-thick) swordfish steaks

2 tablespoons olive oil

1. In a medium bowl, combine cilantro, lime and orange juices and zest, and pineapple. Set aside.
2. Set a gas grill to medium-high, or heat a cast iron skillet over medium-high heat. Mix salt and pepper together in a small bowl.
3. Brush swordfish with oil and sprinkle with salt and pepper mixture.
4. Add fish to grill or skillet, and cook 5 minutes on one side and 3 minutes on other side.
5. Transfer swordfish to plates, top with pineapple salsa, and serve.

Seared Sesame Tuna

With just three ingredients and ready in less than 15 minutes, this low-FODMAP recipe is a beautiful and delicious way to enjoy fish at home.

¾ pound tuna steaks

¼ cup sesame seeds

1 tablespoon garlic-infused olive oil

1. To prepare tuna, discard veiny stub of fish, then slice into 1-inch pieces.
2. Place sesame seeds on a plate and add tuna pieces, tossing to coat all sides with seeds.
3. Heat oil in a 10-inch nonstick frying pan over medium heat. Add tuna, and sear on one side 15–20 seconds. Use tongs to turn tuna, and continue searing all sides of fish. Transfer to a serving plate and serve.

Serves 2	
Per Serving	
Calories	347
Fat	16g
Protein	45g
Sodium	78mg
Fiber	2g
Carbohydrates	4g
Sugar	0g

Bacon-Wrapped Maple Scallops

Easy to prepare, these low-FODMAP scallops make for talk-of-the-party hors d'oeuvres.

20 sea scallops

10 slices bacon, halved

1 recipe Pumpkin Maple Glaze (Chapter 10)

1. Preheat broiler, and line a baking sheet with foil.
2. Wrap each scallop with bacon, securing each with a toothpick. Place on prepared baking sheet.
3. Broil 10–12 minutes, turning once, until bacon is fully cooked on all sides.
4. Drizzle glaze evenly over scallops and serve immediately.

Serves 10	
Per Serving	
Calories	128
Fat	7g
Protein	9g
Sodium	368mg
Fiber	0g
Carbohydrates	6g
Sugar	4g

Salmon with Herbs

The low-FODMAP diet includes many fresh herbs, and this recipe utilizes a few of them. This lovely fish is ready in less than 30 minutes. Serve with a green salad and rice or quinoa.

Serves 4	
Per Serving	
Calories	420
Fat	32g
Protein	23g
Sodium	214mg
Fiber	1g
Carbohydrates	1g
Sugar	2g

1 pound salmon fillets

¼ teaspoon salt

½ teaspoon ground black pepper

¼ cup plus 2 tablespoons olive oil

¼ cup chopped dill

2 tablespoons roughly chopped rosemary leaves

¼ cup flat-leaf parsley leaves

2 tablespoons thyme leaves

2 tablespoons lemon juice

1. Preheat oven to 250°F.
2. Coat a 9" × 13" casserole dish with cooking spray. Lay salmon skin-side down, and sprinkle with salt and pepper.
3. In a food processor, blend oil with dill, rosemary, parsley, thyme, and lemon juice. Use a spatula or your hands to pat the herb paste over the salmon.
4. Bake 22–28 minutes, depending on thickness of salmon. Insert tines of a fork into thickest part of fillet and gently pull. If fish flakes easily, it is done.
5. Slide a spatula under fish and set on a cutting board. Cut into equal pieces and serve.

Mediterranean Flaky Fish with Vegetables

Lovely Mediterranean flavors paired with flaky fish make for a healthy and tasty low-FODMAP dinner. Other great fish options for this recipe are halibut, flounder, red snapper, and tilapia. Pair this dish with a salad and potatoes.

4 (3.5-ounce) skinless Atlantic cod fillets

1 cup grated zucchini

¼ cup thinly sliced basil leaves, plus 4 whole basil leaves

20 cherry tomatoes, halved

10 black olives, sliced

¼ teaspoon kosher salt

½ teaspoon ground black pepper

4 tablespoons dry white wine, divided

4 tablespoons extra-virgin olive oil, divided

Serves 4	
Per Serving	
Calories	209
Fat	12g
Protein	19g
Sodium	261mg
Fiber	2g
Carbohydrates	5g
Sugar	3g

1. Preheat oven to 400°F.
2. Make parchment paper pockets: Pull out a 17" × 11" piece of parchment paper. With one longer edge closest to you, fold in half from left to right. Using scissors, cut out a large heart shape. On a large cutting board or clean work surface, lay down parchment heart and place fish on one half of heart, leaving at least a 1½-inch border around fillet. Repeat with remaining fish fillets.
3. In a medium bowl, combine zucchini, sliced basil, tomatoes, olives, salt, and pepper. Stir to combine.
4. Evenly distribute vegetables among parchment hearts, placing them on top of each fish fillet.
5. Fold each parchment heart in half to close, making edges line up. Starting at rounded end, crimp edges together tightly. Leave a few inches at pointed end unfolded. Grab pointed edge and tilt heart to pour in 1 tablespoon each of wine and oil. Finish by crimping edges and twisting pointed end around and under packet. Lay packets in a 9" × 13" baking dish.
6. Bake until just cooked through, about 10–12 minutes. To test doneness, poke a toothpick through a packet. Fish is done if toothpick easily slides through fish. Carefully cut open packets (steam will escape). Garnish with whole basil leaves and serve.

Basic Baked Scallops

This easy recipe helps the scallops' gentle flavor take center stage. With a satisfying crunch from the gluten-free bread crumb coating, this low-FODMAP dish hits all the right marks. This recipe takes less than 30 minutes to make and pairs well with green beans or a side salad.

Serves 2	
Per Serving	
Calories	516
Fat	28g
Protein	24g
Sodium	1,131mg
Fiber	3g
Carbohydrates	41g
Sugar	2g

¾ pound sea scallops

2 tablespoons lemon juice

2½ tablespoons unsalted butter, melted

¼ teaspoon sea salt

½ teaspoon ground black pepper

2 tablespoons chopped flat-leaf parsley

½ cup gluten-free bread crumbs

½ teaspoon smoked paprika

2 tablespoons olive oil

1. Preheat oven to 425°F.
2. In a 2-quart baking dish, toss together scallops, lemon juice, melted butter, salt, and pepper.
3. In a medium bowl, combine parsley, bread crumbs, paprika, and oil. Sprinkle mixture on top of scallops.
4. Bake 12–14 minutes or until scallops are heated through and bread crumbs are golden. Serve immediately.

Cornmeal-Crusted Tilapia

If you miss fried fish on your low-FODMAP diet, then try this crunchy, flaky fish, using cornmeal made from whole-grain corn. Serve this dish with some lemon wedges and the Tartar Sauce from Chapter 2.

1 pound tilapia fillets

¼ cup gluten-free bread crumbs

¾ cup coarse cornmeal

2 tablespoons gluten-free all-purpose flour

½ teaspoon salt

1 teaspoon ground black pepper

⅛ teaspoon wheat-free asafetida powder

1 large egg

1 tablespoon lactose-free milk

1 tablespoon sunflower oil

1. Rinse fish and pat dry. Slice each fillet into 2 pieces.
2. In a large bowl, combine bread crumbs, cornmeal, flour, salt, pepper, and asafetida. In a small bowl, whisk together egg and milk.
3. Dip tilapia in egg mixture, tapping off any excess. Then dip each side of fish in cornmeal mixture.
4. Heat oil in a 9-inch frying pan over medium-high heat. Pan-fry fish pieces 3–5 minutes each side. Fish should be opaque throughout and flaky when done. Serve.

Serves 4

Per Serving

Calories	228
Fat	7g
Protein	26g
Sodium	260mg
Fiber	1g
Carbohydrates	15g
Sugar	0g

Uses for Cornmeal on the Low-FODMAP Diet

On the low-FODMAP diet, cornmeal is as versatile as it is yummy. This grain makes a gorgeous crispy coating for fish, but it can also be cooked into creamy polenta—which can make a wonderful side dish or an inventive pizza crust (see recipe in Chapter 4).

Fish and Chips

This recipe is healthier than traditional fish and chips, since it bakes the fish and potatoes rather than frying them. But don't worry about the texture: The millet coating adds the familiar crunch of fried fish.

Serves 4	
Per Serving	
Calories	304
Fat	8g
Protein	22g
Sodium	559mg
Fiber	4g
Carbohydrates	35g
Sugar	3g

Corn and the Low-FODMAP Diet

On the low-FODMAP diet, a serving of sweet corn is limited to half of a cob, as eating the whole cob would expose you to high levels of GOS and sorbitol. However, cornmeal, cornstarch, and popcorn are permitted in larger servings, because they're made from a different variety of corn.

¼ cup millet

¼ cup chopped pecans

2 tablespoons coarse cornmeal

1½ teaspoons sea salt, divided

⅛ teaspoon ground red pepper

4 small red potatoes, thinly sliced

1 tablespoon extra-virgin olive oil

½ cup lactose-free milk

2 tablespoons lactose-free sour cream

12 ounces tilapia fillets

1. In a medium bowl, cover millet with boiling water and allow to soak 30 minutes.
2. Preheat oven to 400°F. Line two baking sheets with parchment paper.
3. Drain millet completely, and spread on one baking sheet. Spread pecans on second baking sheet. Roast millet and pecans 10 minutes, tossing halfway through the cooking time.
4. Transfer pecans to a food processor and process until finely ground. In a medium dish, combine ground pecans, millet, cornmeal, ½ teaspoon salt, and red pepper.
5. Reline a baking sheet with parchment paper. In a medium bowl, toss potato slices with oil and remaining 1 teaspoon salt, and scatter potatoes on baking sheet. Roast in oven 30 minutes or until brown and crisp.
6. In a separate medium shallow dish, whisk together milk and sour cream.
7. Reline the second baking sheet with parchment paper and coat with cooking spray. Working with 1 piece at a time, dip tilapia in milk mixture and then carefully coat both sides in millet mixture. Transfer to baking sheet.
8. Bake 15 minutes or until fish is cooked through. Serve potatoes and fish together.

Atlantic Cod with Basil Walnut Sauce

This basil walnut sauce is a lovely complement to cod, and it's just as good with other fish, such as haddock, tilapia, pollack, or striped bass. Serve this dish with your favorite rice, spooning the savory cooking juices over both the fish and the rice.

2 (6-ounce) Atlantic cod fillets

¼ teaspoon kosher salt, divided

½ teaspoon ground black pepper, divided

Zest of 1 large lemon

3 tablespoons extra-virgin olive oil, divided

¼ cup (packed) basil leaves

1 tablespoon small walnut pieces

Serves 2	
Per Serving	
Calories	344
Fat	23g
Protein	31g
Sodium	331mg
Fiber	1g
Carbohydrates	1g
Sugar	0g

1. Preheat oven to 400°F.
2. Place fish fillets in a 9" × 13" baking dish and sprinkle ⅛ teaspoon salt, ¼ teaspoon pepper, and lemon zest over both sides of fish. Brush with 1 tablespoon oil.
3. Using a food processor, combine basil, walnuts, and remaining ⅛ teaspoon salt and ¼ teaspoon pepper. Process until a paste forms. With processor running, gradually add 2 remaining tablespoons oil. Pat mixture evenly over fish.
4. Place baking dish in oven, and bake 13–17 minutes or until fish is opaque in color. Serve.

Baked Moroccan-Style Halibut

This low-FODMAP fish dish was created with a combination of ingredients and spices similar to those used in Moroccan cooking. Easy and flavor-rich, this dish is sure to surprise.

Serves 4

Per Serving

Calories 244
Fat 10g
Protein 32g
Sodium 184mg
Fiber 1g
Carbohydrates 3g
Sugar 2g

1 pint cherry tomatoes

¼ cup pitted black olives

⅛ teaspoon wheat-free asafetida powder

½ teaspoon ground cumin

¼ teaspoon ground cinnamon

¼ teaspoon ground black pepper

4 (6-ounce) halibut fillets

2 tablespoons olive oil

1. Preheat oven to 450°F.
2. In a medium mixing bowl, stir together tomatoes, olives, asafetida, cumin, cinnamon, and pepper.
3. Place halibut in a large baking dish. Sprinkle tomato mixture evenly over fish. Drizzle oil over fish.
4. Bake 10–15 minutes or until an instant-read thermometer inserted into the thickest fillet reads 145°F. Serve immediately.

CHAPTER 7

Vegan and Vegetarian Main Dishes

Mixed Grain and Seed Bowls with Vegetables

These bowls are very nutritious and come with a nice dose of healthy fats, magnesium, and iron, as well as vitamins A, B_6, and C.

Serves 4

Per Serving

Calories	274
Fat	11g
Protein	7g
Sodium	66mg
Fiber	6g
Carbohydrates	38g
Sugar	5g

2 medium sweet potatoes, peeled and cut into 2-inch chunks

2 tablespoons olive oil

1½ tablespoons balsamic vinegar

½ teaspoon dried rosemary

½ teaspoon dried thyme

½ teaspoon dried oregano

2 tablespoons pumpkin seeds

⅔ cup sliced fennel

½ cup brown rice, cooked

¾ cup red quinoa, rinsed and cooked

1 cup buckwheat, rinsed and cooked

½ tablespoon coconut oil

3 cups baby spinach

1. Preheat oven to 375°F.
2. Place sweet potato chunks in a medium bowl. Add oil, vinegar, rosemary, thyme, and oregano. Toss with hands to coat. Place on rimmed baking sheet and roast 45 minutes. Halfway through cooking time, flip potatoes and add pumpkin seeds and fennel.
3. To the same bowl used to prepare sweet potatoes, add rice, quinoa, and buckwheat. Stir in coconut oil.
4. Once sweet potatoes have finished baking and are tender, immediately add to bowl. Add spinach and toss. Divide into four bowls and serve immediately.

Mexican-Style Risotto

Kick your risotto up a notch and try this zesty vegetarian version inspired by traditional Mexican flavors.

½ each large red, green, yellow, and orange bell peppers, seeded and chopped

1 cup frozen corn

¼ teaspoon salt, divided

¼ teaspoon ground black pepper, divided

2 tablespoons salted butter

1 cup Arborio rice

3 cups Vegetable Stock (Chapter 2), divided

1 cup white cooking wine

½ tablespoon ground cumin

2 teaspoons chili powder

1 teaspoon dried oregano

1 teaspoon ground coriander

Juice of 1 large lime

1 cup shredded Cheddar cheese

⅓ cup chopped cilantro

1 medium avocado, peeled, pitted, and cut into sixths

Serves 6

Per Serving

Calories 333
Fat 14g
Protein 9g
Sodium 287mg
Fiber 4g
Carbohydrates 38g
Sugar 2g

1. Coat a small saucepan with cooking spray, and sauté bell peppers over medium-high heat. After about 5 minutes, add corn, and season with ⅛ teaspoon salt and ⅛ teaspoon black pepper. Continue cooking until peppers are slightly charred, about 8 minutes. Set aside.

2. Meanwhile, in a medium skillet over medium-high heat, melt butter. Add rice and fry, stirring, until translucent, about 2 minutes.

3. Slowly add ½ cup stock, and continuously stir until rice has absorbed all liquid. Follow this process again in ½-cup increments until stock is gone, and then add wine in ½-cup increments. Rice should be creamy and tender after 25–35 minutes. If rice is not completely cooked through, add more stock or wine. When cooked through, stir in peppers.

4. In a small bowl, stir together cumin, chili powder, oregano, coriander, lime juice, and remaining ⅛ teaspoon salt and ⅛ teaspoon pepper. Stir into cooked rice, along with Cheddar.

5. Top each serving with some cilantro and 1 slice avocado. Serve immediately.

Lentil Pie

Lentils, Swiss chard, and potatoes make this dish perfect for a chilly day. Maybe you'd like to bring it as a FODMAP-safe dish to your next fall or winter holiday gathering!

Serves 4	
Per Serving	
Calories	513
Fat	15g
Protein	20g
Sodium	1,331mg
Fiber	13g
Carbohydrates	72g
Sugar	6g

1 small sweet potato, peeled and grated

1 small white potato, peeled and grated

2 tablespoons olive oil, divided

4 ounces vegetarian Parmesan cheese, grated

1 medium leek, dark green parts only, finely sliced

1 large carrot, peeled and cut into rounds

1 medium celeriac bulb, peeled and sliced

⅓ cup dry white wine

8 ounces Swiss chard, ribs and stems removed, cut into thin ribbons

2 cups Vegetable Stock (Chapter 2)

1 (15-ounce) can red lentils, thoroughly rinsed and drained

1 medium tomato, diced

½ teaspoon sea salt

1 teaspoon ground black pepper

1. Preheat oven to 350°F. Grease an 8" × 8" ovenproof casserole dish.
2. In a medium bowl, stir together sweet potato, white potato, 1 tablespoon oil, and Parmesan. Set aside.
3. Heat remaining 1 tablespoon oil in a medium nonstick pan over medium-high heat. Add leek leaves, carrots, celeriac, and wine. Cook, covered, 8–10 minutes, stirring occasionally, until vegetables are soft. Add Swiss chard and stock, and bring to a boil, stirring occasionally.
4. Add lentils, tomatoes, salt, and pepper. Stir and cook 5 minutes.
5. Transfer vegetable filling to casserole dish, and top evenly with potato mixture. Bake 20 minutes. Filling should be steaming hot, and potato topping should be golden and cooked through. Serve.

Vegan Cypriot-Style Potato Salad

This low-FODMAP version of traditional Greek Cypriot–style potato salad is a delightful taste of the Mediterranean. If you can't find Cyprus potatoes, you can use Yukon Gold potatoes instead. For a non-vegan version, toss in ¼ cup of feta cheese in the last step.

2½ pounds Cyprus potatoes, peeled

Juice of 1 medium lemon

2 tablespoons extra-virgin olive oil

½ teaspoon sea salt

1 teaspoon ground black pepper

1 tablespoon dried oregano

1 small bunch cilantro, roughly chopped

¼ cup chopped flat-leaf parsley

3 green onions, chopped, green parts only

1 tablespoon olive oil

¼ cup roughly chopped black olives

2 tablespoons capers, rinsed and drained

Serves 6	
Per Serving	
Calories	221
Fat	8g
Protein	3g
Sodium	653mg
Fiber	4g
Carbohydrates	36g
Sugar	2g

1. In a shallow pan of salted boiling water, cook potatoes 25 minutes. Drain and set aside until cool, then slice into small chunks.
2. Place potatoes in a large bowl with lemon juice and extra-virgin olive oil. Add salt, pepper, and oregano. Toss to coat evenly.
3. Add cilantro, parsley, and green onions. Toss to mix.
4. In a small skillet over medium heat, warm olive oil. Add olives and capers, and fry 3 minutes. Sprinkle over potato mixture in bowl. Tastes best when served immediately but can be stored in refrigerator in an airtight container up to 2 days.

Macadamia and Quinoa–Stuffed Peppers

These peppers are a taste and texture adventure. The macadamia nuts add a nice crunch, the avocado a creaminess, and the spices a warming flavor. And the best part is this low-FODMAP dish will keep you feeling full and satisfied for hours. This recipe calls for red bell peppers, but feel free to use green, yellow, or orange if you prefer.

Serves 4	
Per Serving	
Calories	303
Fat	15g
Protein	9g
Sodium	149mg
Fiber	8g
Carbohydrates	34g
Sugar	7g

½ cup quinoa

1 cup Vegetable Stock (Chapter 2)

3 tablespoons nutritional yeast

2 cups whole spinach leaves

2 teaspoons ground cumin

1 tablespoon chili powder

1 cup whole-kernel corn, drained

2 tablespoons macadamia nuts

4 large red bell peppers, tops cut off, seeds removed, halved

2 tablespoons coconut oil

½ medium ripe avocado, peeled, pitted, and sliced into eighths

1 tablespoon fresh lime juice

1. Preheat oven to 375°F. Lightly grease a 9" × 13" baking dish or rimmed baking sheet with cooking spray.
2. In a medium saucepan, combine quinoa with stock. Place over high heat, and bring to a boil. Cover, reduce heat to low, and simmer 15 minutes or until quinoa is tender.
3. Add cooked quinoa to a large mixing bowl, and thoroughly mix together with nutritional yeast, spinach, cumin, chili powder, corn, and macadamia nuts.
4. Place peppers in baking dish, and brush with coconut oil. Stuff peppers with quinoa mixture. Make sure none of the spinach is showing. Cover dish with foil.
5. Bake 30 minutes, then remove foil, increase heat to 400°F, and bake another 30 minutes.
6. Top with avocado, then lime juice. Serve immediately.

Vegetable Nori Roll

Rich and nutty tahini, lemon, and creamy avocado steal the show for this vegan nori roll. These rolls are great for dinner or as appetizers, or they can be made the night before and enjoyed for lunch.

1 perforated half cut (0.08-ounce) nori sheet

½ tablespoon tahini

1 ounce medium tofu, drained, patted dry

2 tablespoons peeled, shredded carrots

1 small cucumber, peeled and thinly sliced

⅛ medium avocado, peeled, pitted, and thinly sliced

Pulp of 1 small lemon slice, cut into thirds

Serves 1	
Per Serving	
Calories	166
Fat	8g
Protein	9g
Sodium	28mg
Fiber	5g
Carbohydrates	18g
Sugar	6g

1. On a bamboo mat, arrange nori sheet horizontally in front of you, rough side facing up.
2. Spread tahini in a horizontal line across bottom half of nori sheet.
3. Spread tofu, carrots, cucumber, avocado, and lemon horizontally across center of tahini.
4. Gently but firmly roll nori around fillings. Dampen outer edge of nori as needed to seal roll.
5. With a sharp knife, carefully slice roll into bite-sized pieces and serve.

Orange Tempeh and Rice Salad

Satisfying, healthy, and easy to make, this low-FODMAP salad can be a meal or can be used as a side to pair with an entrée.

Serves 2

Per Serving

Calories 715
Fat 39g
Protein 19g
Sodium 1,385mg
Fiber 9g
Carbohydrates 72g
Sugar 19g

Tempting Tempeh

Tempeh is a versatile vegan protein. You can use it in salads, sandwiches, curry dishes, stir-fries, tacos, pizza, and more.

Salad

4 tablespoons coconut oil, divided

¾ cup tempeh, cut into small cubes

1½ cups cooked basmati rice

1 cup shredded green cabbage

1 cup broccoli florets

1 cup peeled and shredded carrots

1 cup diced red bell pepper

1 teaspoon ground ginger

1 teaspoon ground cumin

1 teaspoon curry powder

⅛ teaspoon wheat-free asafetida powder

⅛ teaspoon salt

1 teaspoon ground black pepper

½ medium orange, seeds removed, sliced into small pieces

Vinaigrette

Juice of ½ medium orange

2 tablespoons extra-virgin olive oil

2 tablespoons rice wine vinegar

1 tablespoon pure maple syrup

2 teaspoons ground ginger

1 teaspoon salt

1 teaspoon ground black pepper

1. In a large nonstick skillet, heat 1 tablespoon coconut oil over medium-high heat. Add tempeh and sear 1–2 minutes each side. Transfer tempeh to a large bowl and set aside.
2. Add 1 tablespoon coconut oil to skillet, and add rice. Cook, stirring, 2 minutes. Transfer rice to bowl with tempeh and set aside.
3. Add remaining 2 tablespoons coconut oil to skillet along with cabbage, broccoli, carrots, and bell pepper, and stir to combine. Add ginger, cumin, curry powder, asafetida, salt, and black pepper. Stir to evenly coat vegetables. Cook 5 minutes or until softened. Add to bowl with rice and tempeh.
4. Add sliced orange to bowl.
5. To make vinaigrette: Place all vinaigrette ingredients in a medium bowl, and whisk to combine.
6. Pour dressing into bowl with salad ingredients, and toss gently to combine. Serve.

Baked Tofu and Vegetables

Delicious sesame, sweet bok choy, and tofu make for a healthy dish and a happy tummy.

2 (14-ounce) packages extra-firm tofu, pressed between paper towels and patted dry

2 tablespoons toasted sesame oil, divided

2 teaspoons sesame seeds

2½ tablespoons gluten-free soy sauce (tamari), divided

7 cups chopped bok choy (about 8 stalks)

1 small bunch green onions, chopped, green parts only

1 medium red bell pepper, seeded and diced

¼ cup slivered almonds

2 tablespoons rice wine vinegar

Serves 6	
Per Serving	
Calories	287
Fat	18g
Protein	24g
Sodium	492mg
Fiber	5g
Carbohydrates	11g
Sugar	2g

1. Preheat oven to 400°F. Grease a large rimmed baking sheet with cooking spray.
2. Cut tofu into 1-inch pieces, and toss in a large bowl with 1 tablespoon sesame oil, sesame seeds, and 2 tablespoons soy sauce.
3. Spread in a single layer on the prepared baking sheet. Bake tofu on lower rack of oven until browned, 25–30 minutes, flipping once during cooking time.
4. While tofu is baking, heat a large skillet over medium-high heat and coat with remaining 1 tablespoon sesame oil.
5. Add bok choy, green onions, bell pepper, almonds, remaining ½ tablespoon soy sauce, and vinegar. Cook until bok choy is slightly tender, stirring frequently. Transfer to same bowl used to prepare tofu.
6. Once tofu is ready, add to vegetables in bowl, and stir until combined. Divide into four bowls and serve.

Vegetable and Rice Noodle Bowl

This Asian-inspired dish has the taste of garlic without the unsettling effects of the fructans. It's perfect to make on a busy weeknight.

Serves 2
Per Serving
Calories 362
Fat 15g
Protein 6g
Sodium 106mg
Fiber 6g
Carbohydrates 51g
Sugar 9g

Teriyaki Sauce

¼ cup rice wine vinegar

1 tablespoon sesame oil

1 tablespoon light brown sugar

¹⁄₁₆ teaspoon wheat-free asafetida powder

1½ teaspoons peeled, minced ginger

¼ teaspoon red pepper flakes

1 teaspoon ground black pepper

Noodles

1 tablespoon coconut oil

2 cups finely chopped broccoli florets

1 small stalk celery, chopped

2 medium carrots, peeled and shredded

3 ounces rice noodles, cooked and drained

1 green onion, chopped, green parts only

2 teaspoons toasted sesame seeds

1. In a medium bowl, whisk together all sauce ingredients until combined. Set aside.
2. Preheat a wok over medium-high heat. Add oil to coat pan. Add broccoli, celery, carrots, and 2 tablespoons prepared teriyaki sauce. Sauté 8 minutes.
3. Stir drained noodles into wok, along with remaining teriyaki sauce. Cook 3 minutes, and serve immediately, garnished with green onions and sesame seeds.

Turmeric Rice with Cranberries

This Persian-style dish is a tad sweet and nutty—a beautiful pairing of seasonings and embellishments with fluffy basmati rice. Finish this dish with a sprinkle of parsley.

½ cup no-sugar-added dried cranberries

2 cups lukewarm water

1 tablespoon coconut oil

2 tablespoons pine nuts

½ teaspoon ground turmeric

1⁄16 teaspoon wheat-free asafetida powder

½ teaspoon saffron, dissolved in ¼ cup hot water

2 tablespoons light brown sugar

¼ teaspoon sea salt

1 cup cooked basmati rice

Serves 2	
Per Serving	
Calories	272
Fat	11g
Protein	4g
Sodium	199mg
Fiber	3g
Carbohydrates	38g
Sugar	11g

1. Soak cranberries in lukewarm water about 10 minutes to plump. Drain.
2. In a wok or medium skillet over medium-high heat, heat oil and stir in cranberries and pine nuts. Add turmeric, asafetida, saffron water, sugar, and salt, and then reduce heat to low. Cook 7 minutes.
3. Add rice, and stir until evenly coated. Serve immediately.

Savory Baked Tofu

This dish is great accompanied by quinoa or Vegetable Fried Rice (see recipe in this chapter).

Serves 4
Per Serving
Calories 135
Fat 11g
Protein 8g
Sodium 13mg
Fiber 2g
Carbohydrates 3g
Sugar 1g

1 (14-ounce) package firm tofu, drained and patted dry

2 teaspoons paprika

$\frac{1}{16}$ teaspoon wheat-free asafetida powder

2 teaspoons curry powder

2 tablespoons extra-virgin olive oil

1. Preheat oven to 400°F. Lightly grease a 9" × 13" casserole dish.
2. Cut tofu widthwise into ½-inch slices.
3. Lay tofu in the casserole dish. Sprinkle on paprika, asafetida, and curry powder, and drizzle with olive oil. Bake 30 minutes. Serve.

Vegetable Fried Rice

Made with brown rice and chock-full of vegetables, this fried rice is a healthy and flavorful choice. This dish is enjoyable on its own or topped with Savory Baked Tofu (see recipe in this chapter).

1 teaspoon palm sugar

1/16 teaspoon wheat-free asafetida powder

1 tablespoon gluten-free soy sauce (tamari)

1 teaspoon gluten-free vegetarian fish sauce

1 tablespoon rice wine vinegar

2 large eggs

1 tablespoon sesame oil

1/2 medium carrot, peeled and thinly sliced

1/2 medium red bell pepper, seeded and diced

1 large green onion, chopped, green parts only

1 tablespoon peeled, grated ginger

1 cup cooked brown rice

2 cups baby spinach

Serves 2	
Per Serving	
Calories	283
Fat	12g
Protein	11g
Sodium	848mg
Fiber	4g
Carbohydrates	32g
Sugar	5g

Make It Vegan

To make this dish vegan, eliminate the eggs and use vegan fish sauce. You can make your own vegan fish sauce at home or buy it online. If you do find a recipe online, make sure to replace any garlic it calls for with asafetida powder.

1. In a small bowl, combine sugar, asafetida, soy sauce, fish sauce, and vinegar. Stir until sugar is dissolved, and set aside.
2. Whisk eggs in a small bowl. Heat a wok or medium skillet over medium-high heat, and spray with cooking spray. Add eggs to pan and cook 4–5 minutes, folding gently, until cooked but still slightly moist. Slide eggs onto a cutting board and set aside.
3. Add sesame oil to pan, then add carrots and bell pepper. Cook 3 minutes, stirring occasionally.
4. Add green onions to pan, stir, and cook 1 minute. Add ginger and cook 1 more minute.
5. Add rice and cook 2 minutes, stirring. Add soy sauce mixture and continue stirring until absorbed into rice, about 2 minutes.
6. Add spinach and cook until wilted, about 3 minutes. Coarsely chop eggs and stir into rice. Serve.

Tempeh Tacos

In this recipe the moist tempeh and cooked cabbage bring a surprisingly delicious texture and flavor to tacos. Nestled in corn tortillas with a bright and tangy salsa, these tacos are sure to delight.

Serves 4

Per Serving

Calories	386
Fat	17g
Protein	16g
Sodium	599mg
Fiber	9g
Carbohydrates	44g
Sugar	8g

Cabbage and the Low-FODMAP Diet

Though common (green) cabbage is low in FODMAPs at 1 cup per serving, it still might be troublesome for some people with IBS. Cooking the cabbage helps to predigest it, making it easier for some to break it down. Cabbage, like other cruciferous vegetables (raw or cooked), can trigger unpleasant gas and bloating, so be sure to stick to the recommended serving size!

1 (8-ounce) package tempeh

2 small tomatoes, chopped

1 teaspoon chili powder

½ teaspoon ground cumin

3 tablespoons lime juice, divided

4 tablespoons water, divided

1½ tablespoons coconut oil, divided

½ medium green bell pepper, seeded and diced

2 cups diced green cabbage

8 (6-inch) soft corn tortillas, warmed

1½ cups Fiesta Salsa (Chapter 10)

½ medium avocado, peeled, pitted, and cut into eighths

1. Crumble tempeh into a large bowl. Add tomatoes, chili powder, cumin, and 1 tablespoon lime juice. Stir together with 1 tablespoon water. If tempeh mixture seems a little dry, add more water and mix again. Set aside.
2. Heat 1 tablespoon oil in a large skillet over medium-high heat. Add bell pepper and cabbage. Cook 10–12 minutes, stirring occasionally, until tender.
3. Add tempeh mixture, and cook 8 minutes, stirring frequently. Halfway through cooking time, add 1 tablespoon lime juice, 1 tablespoon water, and remaining ½ tablespoon oil. Toward end of cooking, add remaining 2 tablespoons water and remaining 1 tablespoon lime juice, and stir again. Remove from heat. Mixture should be moist—add more water, a tablespoon at a time, if necessary.
4. Fill tortillas with tempeh mixture, salsa, and cooked cabbage mixture. Top with avocado and serve.

Collard Green Wraps with Thai Peanut Dressing

Collard greens are packed with soluble fiber, and they have vitamins C, K, and A, as well as folate, manganese, calcium, and tryptophan—making them a nutrient-dense wrapper for any savory filling. These wraps are bursting with crunchy, colorful ingredients, and along with the dressing they will make for some happy taste buds!

¼ teaspoon salt

2 teaspoons lemon juice

6 large collard green leaves

9 ounces medium-firm tofu, sliced into sticks

⅔ cup bean sprouts

2 medium carrots, peeled and julienned

1 medium cucumber, peeled and julienned

2 tablespoons chopped cilantro leaves

½ small avocado, peeled, pitted, and cut into 6 slices

Thai Peanut Dressing (Chapter 10)

Serves 3	
Per Serving	
Calories	342
Fat	17g
Protein	15g
Sodium	1,148mg
Fiber	7g
Carbohydrates	36g
Sugar	23g

1. Set a wide saucepan over high heat, and fill it with 3 inches of water. Add salt and lemon juice. Bring water to a simmer, and reduce heat to medium. Place 1 collard green leaf in water until it turns bright green, 35–45 seconds, then remove from water and place on a plate with paper towels to cool. Repeat with each leaf.
2. Place 1½ ounces tofu toward top of each collard green leaf. Top each with equal amounts of sprouts, carrots, cucumber, cilantro, and avocado. Drizzle Thai Peanut Dressing over vegetables.
3. Roll wraps up burrito-style, tucking in sides as you roll. Slice each roll in half, and serve.

CHAPTER 8

Vegetables and Sides

Herbed Mashed Potatoes

Simply luscious, these potatoes are great on their own or paired with beef or fish. Serve them with an added pat of butter on top to kick up the creamy, delicious flavor.

Serves 4
Per Serving
Calories 188
Fat 6g
Protein 3g
Sodium 371mg
Fiber 4g
Carbohydrates 32g
Sugar 2g

1½ pounds Yukon Gold potatoes, peeled and cut into quarters

½ teaspoon salt

1 tablespoon lactose-free milk

2 tablespoons unsalted butter

⅟₁₆ teaspoon wheat-free asafetida powder

½ tablespoon dried oregano

½ tablespoon dried thyme

½ tablespoon dried rosemary

½ tablespoon ground black pepper

1. Heat a large saucepan or pot over high heat.
2. Add potatoes, salt, and enough cold water to cover potatoes. Once boiling, reduce heat to low, cover, and cook about 15 minutes. When potatoes are tender, drain and return to pot.
3. Add milk and butter, and start to mash with potato masher. After about 1 minute of mashing, add asafetida, oregano, thyme, rosemary, and pepper. Continue mashing to desired consistency. Serve.

Swiss Chard with Pine Nuts and Parmesan

This mild side dish is packed with nutrients and goes very well with fish. If you're watching your sodium intake, you can lower the amount in this dish significantly by simply skipping the salt. The Parmesan provides most of the remaining sodium, along with a lovely final flavor.

2 tablespoons unsalted butter

2 tablespoons garlic-infused olive oil

1 bunch Swiss chard, ribs and stems removed and chopped together, leaves coarsely chopped separately

½ cup dry white wine

1 tablespoon fresh lemon juice

3 tablespoons pine nuts

1⁄16 teaspoon sea salt

2 tablespoons grated Parmesan cheese

½ teaspoon ground black pepper

Serves 4	
Per Serving	
Calories	181
Fat	16g
Protein	2g
Sodium	128mg
Fiber	1g
Carbohydrates	3g
Sugar	1g

1. Heat butter and oil in a large skillet set over medium-high heat.
2. Add chard ribs and stems and wine, and simmer until ribs and stems begin to soften, about 5 minutes.
3. Stir in chard leaves, and cook until wilted.
4. Stir in lemon juice and pine nuts, and cook about 30 seconds. Add salt.
5. Using tongs, transfer half of mixture to a serving plate. Add 1 tablespoon Parmesan, then remaining mixture, then remaining 1 tablespoon Parmesan. Top with pepper and serve.

Herbed Yellow Squash

This dish is best made when squash are in season. A little butter and some herbs make this side dish delicious.

Serves 2	
Per Serving	
Calories	111
Fat	6g
Protein	5g
Sodium	530mg
Fiber	4g
Carbohydrates	13g
Sugar	8g

1 tablespoon unsalted butter

1½ pounds yellow squash, cut into ¼-inch circles

½ cup chicken broth

3 sprigs thyme

1 tablespoon chopped rosemary

¼ teaspoon salt

2 tablespoons chopped flat-leaf parsley

½ teaspoon ground black pepper

1. Heat butter in a small skillet over medium-high heat. Add squash and sauté about 1 minute.
2. Add broth, thyme, rosemary, and salt, and bring to a simmer.
3. Partially cover and reduce heat to low. Cook until tender, about 6–8 minutes, stirring occasionally.
4. Add parsley and pepper and serve.

Coconut Rice

This flavorful rice would complement a stir-fry, a Thai-style soup, or a simple roasted chicken or fish.

1 tablespoon coconut oil

½ teaspoon peeled, grated ginger

2 cups cooked jasmine rice

1 (13.5-ounce) can coconut milk

¼ cup shredded unsweetened coconut

¼ teaspoon Himalayan salt

1 tablespoon lime juice

Serves 2	
Per Serving	
Calories	708
Fat	51g
Protein	9g
Sodium	221mg
Fiber	3g
Carbohydrates	53g
Sugar	1g

1. In a 6-inch skillet, heat oil over medium heat. Once oil is shimmering, add ginger and cook 2–3 minutes.
2. Add rice, coconut milk, coconut, and salt. Cook and stir until rice mixture is heated through, 5–7 minutes.
3. Stir in lime juice and remove from heat. Serve.

Garlicky Parsnip and Carrot Fries

These fries are a surprising take on the traditional French fry—and they're more nutritious too! They make a fun and delicious treat for a family meal or a party.

Serves 6

Per Serving

Calories	98
Fat	5g
Protein	1g
Sodium	200mg
Fiber	4g
Carbohydrates	14g
Sugar	5g

2 tablespoons garlic-infused olive oil

⅛ teaspoon wheat-free asafetida powder

2 teaspoons chopped flat-leaf parsley

½ teaspoon coarse salt

5 medium carrots, peeled and cut diagonally into 1-inch slices

3 medium parsnips, peeled and cut diagonally into 1-inch slices

1. Preheat oven to 400°F.
2. In a large bowl, combine oil, asafetida, parsley, and salt. Add carrots and parsnips to bowl, and toss well to coat.
3. Place on a rimmed baking sheet and roast 20 minutes, flipping pieces halfway through roasting time. When parsnips and carrots are crisp and golden brown, remove from oven and serve.

Potato and Kale Gratin

This warm and cheesy dish makes for a satisfying, comforting meal, and it's also great for the holidays.

2 tablespoons unsalted butter, cut into small pieces, plus more for buttering pan

1 large bunch (about ½ pound) kale, chopped (ribs and stems removed)

½ cup lactose-free milk

1 teaspoon sea salt

½ teaspoon ground black pepper

1 pound Yukon Gold potatoes, very thinly sliced

½ cup grated Parmesan cheese, divided

1 tablespoon thyme leaves

Serves 4	
Per Serving	
Calories	239
Fat	10g
Protein	9g
Sodium	660mg
Fiber	5g
Carbohydrates	28g
Sugar	4g

1. Preheat oven to 400°F, and place a rack in middle of oven. Butter a 9" × 13" baking dish.
2. Bring a large pot of water to a boil and add kale. Boil 2–3 minutes or until leaves are wilted. Drain in a colander, squeezing out excess water. Set aside.
3. In a medium bowl, whisk together milk, salt, and pepper. Set aside.
4. Layer about half of potato slices evenly on bottom of baking dish. Top with kale, then with ¼ cup Parmesan. Layer remaining potatoes on top, and sprinkle with remaining ¼ cup Parmesan.
5. Pour milk mixture over potatoes. Sprinkle with thyme leaves, and scatter butter pieces on top.
6. Bake, covered with aluminum foil, 25 minutes. Remove foil and bake another 25 minutes or until potatoes are tender and cheese is golden brown. Serve.

Swiss Chard with Cranberries and Pine Nuts

This recipe was inspired by a Sicilian dish that traditionally includes spinach, currants, and pine nuts. Cranberries are allowed on the low-FODMAP diet, and it's best to use ones without added sugar.

Serves 4	
Per Serving	
Calories	130
Fat	7g
Protein	6g
Sodium	607mg
Fiber	5g
Carbohydrates	12g
Sugar	4g

2½ pounds Swiss chard

1 tablespoon garlic-infused olive oil

3 tablespoons pine nuts

⅛ teaspoon wheat-free asafetida powder

3 tablespoons no-sugar-added dried cranberries

1/16 teaspoon salt

¼ teaspoon ground black pepper

1. Fill a medium bowl with ice water. Bring a large pot of salted water to a boil. Add chard, and cook until tender, about 2 minutes. Transfer chard to ice water, and let sit 5 minutes. Drain in a colander, and squeeze out as much water as possible. Remove stems and ribs, and chop leaves coarsely.
2. In a large, heavy skillet or cast iron pan, heat oil over medium heat.
3. Add pine nuts and asafetida, and cook 2–3 minutes.
4. Add chard and cranberries, and cook until heated through, 2–3 minutes. Season with salt and pepper. Serve.

Zoodles with Pesto

Making "zoodles," or zucchini noodles, is not only fun—it's also a vegetable-forward way to enjoy wheat-free pasta.

1 tablespoon extra-virgin olive oil

1 pound zucchini, cut into long, thin noodles with a spiral slicer or vegetable peeler

1/16 teaspoon sea salt

1/8 teaspoon ground black pepper

1 1/8 cups Pesto Sauce (Chapter 2)

1. Heat olive oil in a medium sauté pan over medium heat.
2. Add zucchini noodles, salt, and pepper, and stir 3–5 minutes or until noodles are just tender.
3. Serve noodles and sauce separately for individual serving, or toss together for a more consistent feel.

Serves 3	
Per Serving	
Calories	368
Fat	33g
Protein	8g
Sodium	423mg
Fiber	2g
Carbohydrates	9g
Sugar	4g

Green Beans with Lemon Pepper

These fragrant, delicate green beans go nicely with meat or fish and are easy to make.

Serves 6	
Per Serving	
Calories	82
Fat	6g
Protein	2g
Sodium	93mg
Fiber	3g
Carbohydrates	6g
Sugar	3g

1 pound fresh green beans, trimmed

2 tablespoons unsalted butter

¼ cup sliced almonds

2 teaspoons lemon pepper

⅛ teaspoon salt

1. Place green beans in a large pot of salted boiling water. Cook until just tender, about 4–5 minutes, and then drain.
2. Meanwhile, melt butter in a large skillet over medium heat. Add almonds and sauté until lightly browned. Sprinkle in lemon pepper and salt. Add green beans and toss to coat. Serve.

Hasselback Potatoes

Hasselback potatoes can be made with different ingredients, but the distinguishing quality is the way they are sliced. Unlike in more traditional recipes, there's no heavy cream here—just lactose-free milk and sour cream, plus cheese. A rimmed baking sheet works for cooking these potatoes in a pinch, but a baking dish or roasting pan is a better option (the smaller size and higher sides keep the potatoes in place).

6 medium baking potatoes

4 tablespoons unsalted butter, melted, divided

1 teaspoon paprika

1/8 teaspoon sea salt

1 teaspoon ground black pepper

2 cups lactose-free milk

2 cups lactose-free sour cream

3 tablespoons finely grated pecorino-style cheese

1 cup gluten-free panko

1 teaspoon dried oregano

Serves 6	
Per Serving	
Calories	521
Fat	24g
Protein	12g
Sodium	430mg
Fiber	5g
Carbohydrates	69g
Sugar	11g

1. Preheat oven to 425°F.
2. Use a sharp knife to make slices 1/4 inch apart across each potato, not slicing all the way through but leaving about 1/8 inch of potato uncut at the bottom.
3. Place potatoes, sliced sides up, in a small roasting pan or a shallow baking dish.
4. Drizzle potatoes with 2 tablespoons melted butter, then sprinkle with paprika, salt, and pepper.
5. Whisk milk and sour cream in a medium bowl, and pour over potatoes.
6. In a small bowl, combine cheese, panko, and oregano. Sprinkle this mixture over top of potatoes, and drizzle with remaining 2 tablespoons butter.
7. Place potatoes in oven and cook 35–45 minutes. When done, potatoes should be cooked through, crispy, and golden brown. Serve hot.

Sesame and Ginger Bok Choy

This side dish is great when paired with Seared Sesame Tuna (Chapter 6). For a vegan meal, try it with brown rice and Savory Baked Tofu (Chapter 7).

Serves 2	
Per Serving	
Calories	103
Fat	7g
Protein	4g
Sodium	597mg
Fiber	3g
Carbohydrates	9g
Sugar	3g

1 tablespoon sesame oil

½ tablespoon peeled, minced ginger

1 green onion, chopped, green parts only

½ cup sliced water chestnuts

4 cups chopped bok choy

1 tablespoon gluten-free soy sauce (tamari)

1. Heat oil in a large skillet over medium heat. Add ginger and green onions, and cook 1 minute.
2. Add water chestnuts, bok choy, and soy sauce, and cook 3–5 minutes or until bok choy greens are wilted and stalks are crisp-tender. Serve.

Spaghetti Squash with Goat Cheese

Spaghetti squash is a low-calorie food and is often used as a wheat-free substitute for pasta. It has a mild nutty flavor and is also high in several vitamins and minerals. Here it's combined with goat cheese to make a light and earthy dish that fares well alongside fish.

1 (5-pound) spaghetti squash

½ cup water

½ tablespoon extra-virgin olive oil

2 tablespoons pine nuts

⅛ teaspoon salt

½ teaspoon ground black pepper

1 ounce crumbled goat cheese

Serves 4	
Per Serving	
Calories	137
Fat	7g
Protein	4g
Sodium	147mg
Fiber	4g
Carbohydrates	17g
Sugar	7g

1. Preheat oven to 400°F.
2. Carefully cut squash in half, and use a spoon to scoop out seeds. (If desired, keep seeds to roast in oven at a later date.) Arrange squash halves cut-side down in a 9" × 13" baking dish. Pour water into dish, and bake until tender, about 30 minutes.
3. With a fork, use a raking motion to pull up the squash's fleshy, noodle-like strands and place them in a large bowl.
4. To the squash, add oil, pine nuts, salt, and pepper. Finish by topping with goat cheese crumbles. Serve immediately.

Potato Soup

Filling and hearty, this soup is great for a cold day. For an attractive and yummy presentation, top each bowl with some additional Cheddar cheese and sliced green onions.

Serves 4	
Per Serving	
Calories	865
Fat	38g
Protein	32g
Sodium	968mg
Fiber	5g
Carbohydrates	90g
Sugar	20g

6 medium russet potatoes, peeled and cut into cubes

¼ cup unsalted butter

½ cup gluten-free all-purpose flour

6 cups lactose-free milk, divided

⅛ teaspoon salt

¼ teaspoon cracked black pepper

¼ pound grated Cheddar cheese

¼ pound grated Parmesan cheese

1 green onion, chopped, green parts only

1. Boil potato cubes in a large pot until tender, about 15 minutes. Drain, add to a food processor, and blend until smooth.
2. In a large saucepan, melt butter over medium heat. Add flour and cook about 1 minute, stirring continuously.
3. Add 3 cups milk to pan with salt and pepper, and stir until there are no lumps. Add remaining 3 cups milk, and increase heat to medium-high. Bring to a rolling boil, stirring constantly.
4. After boiling, turn heat off and add blended potatoes, cheeses, and green onion. Stir until cheeses are melted. Serve immediately in soup bowls.

Carrot and Ginger Soup

This elegant soup is sure to soothe your whole system. For a vegetarian version, feel free to substitute Vegetable Stock (see recipe in Chapter 2).

2 tablespoons pumpkin seeds

2 tablespoons extra-virgin olive oil

1 pound carrots, peeled and thinly sliced

1 (2-inch) piece ginger, peeled and grated

4 cups Easy Onion- and Garlic-Free Chicken Stock (Chapter 2)

2 teaspoons grated orange zest

¼ cup fresh orange juice

⅛ teaspoon sea salt

⅛ teaspoon ground black pepper

Serves 6	
Per Serving	
Calories	104
Fat	6g
Protein	4g
Sodium	91mg
Fiber	2g
Carbohydrates	9g
Sugar	5g

1. Preheat broiler. On a rimmed baking sheet, toast pumpkin seeds until golden brown, about 3 minutes. Set aside.
2. Heat oil in a large stockpot over medium-low heat. Add carrots and ginger, and sauté 5 minutes, stirring frequently.
3. Add stock. Turn heat to high and bring just to a boil, then lower heat and simmer, uncovered, 20 minutes or until carrots are soft.
4. Purée mixture in a blender or food processor. Return to pot. Stir in orange zest and juice, salt, and pepper.
5. Serve soup in bowls, garnished with pumpkin seeds.

Lentil Chili

Who says you can't enjoy a little chili? This chili replaces high-FODMAP beans with canned lentils. If you don't have the time or energy to dice a large carrot, you can substitute a cup of store-bought shredded carrots.

Serves 4	
Per Serving	
Calories	294
Fat	11g
Protein	9g
Sodium	411mg
Fiber	9g
Carbohydrates	43g
Sugar	6g

1 tablespoon olive oil

1 medium stalk celery, diced

1 large carrot, peeled and diced

1 large red bell pepper, seeded and chopped

4 cups Vegetable Stock (Chapter 2), divided

2 teaspoons chili powder

1 teaspoon ground cumin

2 cups canned lentils, drained and thoroughly rinsed

3 medium Roma tomatoes, diced

¼ cup chopped cilantro

2 cups baby spinach

½ cup lactose-free sour cream

1. Heat a large pot over medium-high heat and add oil. Once hot, add celery, carrots, and bell pepper. Sauté about 5 minutes, stirring frequently, until vegetables are tender.
2. Stir in ¼ cup stock. Add chili powder and cumin and stir. Cook 1 minute.
3. Add lentils, tomatoes, cilantro, and remaining 3¾ cups stock. Once boiling, reduce heat to medium-low and simmer 25 minutes, partially covered.
4. Uncover and cook 8 minutes longer. Add spinach and stir while cooking another 2 minutes.
5. Ladle into bowls, top with sour cream, and serve.

Greek Pasta Salad

When you need a little Greek food fix, this pasta salad will do the trick! This recipe is great for a barbecues or a make-ahead lunch. It can be made ahead and kept, covered, in the refrigerator for up to 1 day.

1 (12-ounce) package spiral-shaped gluten-free rice pasta

¼ cup garlic-infused olive oil

¼ cup extra-virgin olive oil

Juice of 1 large lemon

⅓ cup rice wine vinegar

2 teaspoons dried oregano

⅛ teaspoon sea salt

¼ teaspoon ground black pepper

1 (10-ounce) bag fresh spinach, rinsed, drained, and coarsely chopped

8 ounces feta cheese, crumbled

1 pint grape tomatoes, halved

½ cup pitted kalamata olives

Serves 6	
Per Serving	
Calories	495
Fat	30g
Protein	12g
Sodium	584mg
Fiber	4g
Carbohydrates	50g
Sugar	3g

1. Cook pasta according to package directions, then drain, rinse, and set aside.
2. Make dressing: In a large bowl, whisk together oils, lemon juice, vinegar, oregano, salt, and pepper.
3. Add spinach, feta, tomatoes, and olives to the bowl.
4. Add pasta, and toss gently until everything is combined and evenly coated. Serve.

Fennel Pomegranate Salad

You will love all the flavors in this salad, from the burst of tartness in the pomegranate seeds, to the mellow bite of fennel and goat cheese, to the tangy lemon juice and earthy olive oil—this salad has it all!

Serves 2

Per Serving

Calories	430
Fat	35g
Protein	9g
Sodium	489mg
Fiber	7g
Carbohydrates	21g
Sugar	12g

Can You Have Pomegranates?

Pomegranates are low in FODMAPs at ¼ cup of seeds per serving. They're also a good source of vitamin C, vitamin K, and dietary fiber.

3 small fennel bulbs, thinly sliced

¼ medium stalk celery, sliced into thin slivers

½ cup coarsely chopped parsley

½ cup pomegranate seeds, divided

¼ cup fresh lemon juice

¼ cup extra-virgin olive oil

¼ teaspoon salt

½ teaspoon ground black pepper

½ cup crumbled goat cheese

1. To a large bowl, add fennel, celery, parsley, and ¼ cup pomegranate seeds. Toss to combine.
2. Add lemon juice and oil, and toss to coat. Add salt and pepper and toss again.
3. Serve topped with goat cheese and remaining ¼ cup pomegranate seeds.

Orange, Red, and Green Buckwheat Salad

Colorful, flavorful, and full of the nutrients your body needs, this salad makes a great lunch, and it's pretty enough to share at a holiday gathering.

2 tablespoons pure maple syrup

2 tablespoons rice wine vinegar

1 tablespoon balsamic vinegar

¼ cup extra-virgin olive oil

¼ teaspoon sea salt

2 cups cooked, rinsed, and cooled buckwheat

½ pound sweet potatoes, peeled, roasted, cooled, and cubed

2 tablespoons no-sugar-added dried cranberries

2 cups arugula

2 cups mesclun greens (a.k.a. spring mix)

¼ cup slivered almonds

1. In a small bowl, whisk together syrup, vinegars, oil, and salt. Set aside.
2. In a large bowl, combine buckwheat, sweet potatoes, cranberries, arugula, mesclun greens, and almonds. Drizzle with dressing and toss gently. Serve.

Serves 4

Per Serving

Calories	324
Fat	17g
Protein	6g
Sodium	137mg
Fiber	6g
Carbohydrates	39g
Sugar	12g

Buckwheat Is Wheat-Free!

Contrary to its name, buckwheat is in fact wheat-free and can be enjoyed on the low-FODMAP diet and gluten-free diets. It's one of the few plant-based foods that contain all nine essential amino acids. Amino acids are the building blocks of proteins; they're important throughout the body. The human body makes some amino acids, but these nine can only be found in foods.

Kale, Fennel, and Blueberry Salad

This salad is a low-FODMAP phytonutrient and vitamin powerhouse! It's also very easy to make, and it can be kept, covered, in the refrigerator for up to 3 days.

Serves 5

Per Serving

Calories	163
Fat	11g
Protein	4g
Sodium	197mg
Fiber	4g
Carbohydrates	15g
Sugar	6g

9 large leaves curly kale, ribs and stems removed, thinly shredded

½ teaspoon sea salt

3 tablespoons extra-virgin olive oil, divided

Juice of 1 large lemon

1 cup shredded butter lettuce

1 medium stalk celery, diced

1 medium yellow bell pepper, seeded and diced

1 medium carrot, peeled and grated

1 tablespoon hemp seeds

1 tablespoon pumpkin seeds

1 tablespoon chopped walnuts

2 cups shredded green cabbage

2 medium radishes, sliced very thin

1 cup sliced fennel

1 cup blueberries

1. Add kale to a large bowl, and sprinkle with salt and 2 tablespoons oil. Massage leaves with hands until leaves begin to darken and soften.
2. Add remaining 1 tablespoon oil and remaining ingredients and toss gently. Serve.

Beef Soup with Buckwheat

This comforting soup takes a little less than an hour to whip up and is very easy to make.

1¼ pounds stew beef

4 quarts Easy Onion- and Garlic-Free Chicken Stock (Chapter 2)

¾ teaspoon paprika

¾ teaspoon gluten-free Worcestershire sauce

3 bay leaves

⅛ teaspoon salt

½ teaspoon ground black pepper

1 cup buckwheat groats

2 large yellow potatoes, diced

1 tablespoon olive oil

2 large carrots, peeled and diced

½ medium stalk celery, diced

¼ cup chopped dill

Serves 4	
Per Serving	
Calories	569
Fat	15g
Protein	54g
Sodium	247mg
Fiber	10g
Carbohydrates	64g
Sugar	4g

1. Place meat in a large pot with stock. Add paprika, Worcestershire, bay leaves, salt, and pepper. Bring to a boil, and then turn heat to medium and cook 40 minutes, uncovered.
2. Add buckwheat and potatoes, and cook until tender, about 15 minutes.
3. In the meantime, in a medium skillet over medium heat, warm oil. Add carrots and celery, and sauté until carrots are softened, about 6–8 minutes. Add to soup, and simmer an additional 5 minutes.
4. Remove bay leaves, add dill to soup, ladle into bowls, and serve.

Carrot, Leek, and Saffron Soup

This type of soup would usually call for heavy cream, but this recipe uses luscious coconut cream instead for a hearty low-FODMAP soup. If you prefer a lighter soup, replace the coconut cream with full-fat coconut milk. For a vegan version, replace the butter with oil.

Serves 4

Per Serving

Calories	257
Fat	18g
Protein	3g
Sodium	178mg
Fiber	6g
Carbohydrates	23g
Sugar	8g

Making Coconut Cream

If you don't have coconut cream on hand, here's how to make it: Chill a can of coconut milk in the refrigerator for 24 hours or more. Open the can carefully, without shaking it. The thick cream on top is your coconut cream. Scoop it out, and keep the liquid at the bottom of the can for another purpose (Chapter 11).

2 tablespoons unsalted butter

2 medium leeks, dark green parts only, coarsely chopped

1 medium red bell pepper, seeded and diced

1 pound carrots, peeled and sliced

1 tablespoon ground coriander

¼ teaspoon cayenne pepper

½ teaspoon ground turmeric

1 teaspoon saffron, divided

4 cups Vegetable Stock (Chapter 2)

⅛ teaspoon salt

¼ teaspoon white pepper

½ cup coconut cream

1. Melt butter in a medium saucepan over medium heat. Add leek leaves and cook 7 minutes or until very soft.
2. Add bell pepper and carrots, and cook another 5–7 minutes or until carrots soften just slightly.
3. Add coriander, cayenne, turmeric, and ½ teaspoon saffron. Stir and cook 1 minute. Add stock, salt, and pepper, and bring to a boil. Reduce heat to low and cover. Cook 20–35 minutes or until vegetables are very tender.
4. Remove soup from heat and let cool to room temperature. Using a blender or food processor, purée soup in batches.
5. Serve in soup bowls, garnishing each with a swirl of cream and a few threads of remaining ½ teaspoon saffron.

Warm Basil and Walnut Potato Salad

Making steak or chicken? Going to a barbecue? Try this fancier (and low-FODMAP) version of potato salad and impress yourself and your friends. If you can't get your hands on Yukon Golds, you can use any variety of yellow potatoes.

¼ cup (packed) basil leaves

1 tablespoon small walnut pieces

⅛ teaspoon kosher salt

½ teaspoon ground black pepper

1½ tablespoons extra-virgin olive oil

4 medium Yukon Gold potatoes, peeled

Zest of 1 medium lemon

Serves 4	
Per Serving	
Calories	201
Fat	6g
Protein	3g
Sodium	462mg
Fiber	4g
Carbohydrates	34g
Sugar	2g

1. In a food processor, combine basil, walnuts, salt, and pepper. Process until a paste forms. With processor running, gradually add oil. Set aside.
2. Place potatoes in a medium pot. Add enough salted water to cover tops of potatoes.
3. Bring water to a boil over medium-high heat, and cook until potatoes are tender, about 15 minutes. A knife inserted into a potato should pierce through easily. Drain, transfer to a cutting board, and cut into chunks.
4. Place potatoes in a large serving bowl and pour on basil-walnut sauce. Toss gently to coat, and add lemon zest. Serve immediately, or cover and refrigerate up to 3 days.

Chicken Salad

This low-FODMAP chicken salad tastes just like home. Serve this on a bed of greens or as a sandwich, or just eat it out of the bowl—it's that yummy!

Serves 4	
Per Serving	
Calories	531
Fat	40g
Protein	40g
Sodium	324mg
Fiber	0g
Carbohydrates	1g
Sugar	0g

1½ pounds boneless, skinless chicken breasts

2 cups Easy Onion- and Garlic-Free Chicken Stock (Chapter 2)

⅛ teaspoon salt, divided

½ teaspoon dried thyme

1 cup Basic Mayonnaise (Chapter 2)

½ medium stalk celery, diced

1½ teaspoons finely chopped tarragon

¼ teaspoon ground black pepper

1. In a 2–4-quart saucepan with a lid, arrange chicken breasts in a single layer. Set pan over medium-high heat, and pour in stock, ¹⁄₁₆ teaspoon salt, and thyme. If stock doesn't cover chicken breasts completely, add water as needed.
2. Bring to a boil, then reduce heat to low and cover pot. Poach chicken 8–12 minutes. Chicken is ready when an instant-read thermometer placed in thickest part of meat registers 165°F. The meat should be opaque throughout. With a slotted spoon, transfer chicken to a plate. Cover and chill in refrigerator 30 minutes.
3. Cut chicken into cubes, removing any excess fat.
4. To a medium bowl, add chicken, mayonnaise, celery, tarragon, remaining ¹⁄₁₆ teaspoon salt, and pepper. Stir well to combine. Chill in refrigerator until ready to serve.

Lemon Kale Salad

Light, lemony, and fresh, this salad is great for lunch—on its own or served alongside an entrée.

10 ounces kale, ribs and stems removed, coarsely chopped

¼ teaspoon sea salt

½ cup extra-virgin olive oil

½ teaspoon ground black pepper

Juice of 2 medium lemons

¼ cup slivered almonds

Serves 4	
Per Serving	
Calories	315
Fat	30g
Protein	5g
Sodium	124mg
Fiber	4g
Carbohydrates	9g
Sugar	2g

1. Place kale in a large bowl. Add salt and oil, and massage with hands until kale becomes soft.
2. Add pepper, lemon juice, and almonds. Toss well to combine. Serve.

Filet Mignon Salad

Grilled filet mignon, probably the most tender and beloved cut of beef, is dressed to the nines in greens, tomatoes, and goat cheese in this salad.

Serves 2

Per Serving

Calories	865
Fat	72g
Protein	37g
Sodium	584mg
Fiber	4g
Carbohydrates	13g
Sugar	7g

¼ large head romaine lettuce, chopped (stem removed)

½ large head Belgian endive, thinly sliced crosswise (about 1½ cups)

¼ cup chopped basil

1½ cups baby arugula

2 teaspoons pure maple syrup

½ cup rice wine vinegar

1½ tablespoons lemon juice

½ teaspoon sea salt

½ teaspoon ground black pepper

½ cup plus ½ tablespoon olive oil, divided

1 tablespoon unsalted butter

½ pound filet mignon

2 ounces crumbled goat cheese

8 cherry tomatoes, halved

1. In a large bowl, combine romaine, endive, basil, and arugula.
2. To a food processor or blender, add syrup, vinegar, lemon juice, salt, and pepper. With machine running on low speed, slowly blend in ½ cup oil. Set aside.
3. In a medium cast iron skillet or stainless steel skillet over medium heat, melt butter with remaining ½ tablespoon oil. Add filet mignon and cook 5–7 minutes on each side (or longer, depending on desired degree of doneness). Allow to stand 5 minutes. Slice into strips of medium thickness.
4. Add filet mignon, goat cheese, and tomatoes to salad bowl. Pour on dressing. Toss well to coat, and serve.

CHAPTER 10

Condiments, Sauces, and Dressings

Vanilla Maple Almond Butter

This almond butter tastes good on top of bananas, in smoothies, on crackers, or with jam! Store this butter in an airtight container in the refrigerator for 6–8 weeks, or freeze for up to 4 months.

Makes 2 cups	
Per Serving **(Serving size: 2 tablespoons)**	
Calories	118
Fat	9g
Protein	4g
Sodium	12mg
Fiber	2g
Carbohydrates	6g
Sugar	2g

2 cups raw almonds

2 tablespoons pure maple syrup

3 teaspoons coconut oil at room temperature, divided

½ teaspoon ground cinnamon

1 teaspoon alcohol-free vanilla extract

⅛ teaspoon sea salt

1. Preheat oven to 350°F.
2. Place almonds on a rimmed baking sheet and toss with syrup and 2 teaspoons coconut oil. Roast about 30 minutes, stirring halfway through cooking time. Allow to cool 10–15 minutes.
3. Place roasted almonds in food processor and process until smooth, about 5 minutes. Stop when needed to scrape down sides.
4. Add cinnamon, vanilla, salt, and remaining 1 teaspoon coconut oil. Process until well combined. Serve.

Toasted Coconut Butter

If you love the flavor of coconut, now you can add it to your smoothie or spread it on your gluten-free bread or bagel, or fruit! This butter can be stored at room temperature for up to 1 year.

1 pound shredded unsweetened coconut

1 teaspoon ground cinnamon

1. Preheat oven to 350°F.
2. Spread coconut evenly on a rimmed baking sheet. Bake 8 minutes or until light golden brown; stir occasionally. Alternately, place coconut shreds in a medium skillet and toast over medium heat, stirring frequently until golden brown.
3. Add toasted coconut and cinnamon to a food processor, and blend on high speed 4–6 minutes or until the consistency of nut butter. Before each use, stir well with a spoon.

Makes 2 cups
Per Serving
(Serving size: 2 tablespoons)
Calories 189
Fat 17g
Protein 2g
Sodium 0mg
Fiber 6g
Carbohydrates 8g
Sugar 2g

Basil Sauce

Use this sauce on top of fish or chicken, or use it to replace the sauce in the Salmon Cakes with Fresh Dill Sauce recipe in Chapter 6 for a new twist on that dish. You can store this sauce in an airtight container in the refrigerator for 5–7 days or in the freezer for 3–4 months.

Makes 1 cup

Per Serving
(Serving size: 1 tablespoon)

Calories	82
Fat	8g
Protein	1g
Sodium	27mg
Fiber	0g
Carbohydrates	1g
Sugar	0g

¼ cup tahini

¼ cup flat-leaf parsley leaves

¼ cup coarsely chopped chives

1 cup (packed) basil leaves

Juice of 2 medium lemons

¼ cup olive oil

¼ teaspoon sea salt

¼ teaspoon ground black pepper

Add all ingredients to a food processor. Blend until smooth. Serve.

Burger Sauce

Change up your burger with this awesome low-FODMAP approved sauce! You can store this sauce in an airtight container in the refrigerator for up to 2 weeks.

Makes 1 cup

Per Serving
(Serving size: 1 tablespoon)

Calories	51
Fat	5g
Protein	1g
Sodium	99mg
Fiber	0g
Carbohydrates	2g
Sugar	1g

2 tablespoons relish

½ cup Basic Mayonnaise (Chapter 2)

¼ cup Artisanal Ketchup (Chapter 2)

1 teaspoon paprika

1 tablespoon Dijon mustard

1 teaspoon ground black pepper

1/16 teaspoon wheat-free asafetida powder

Stir together all ingredients in a medium bowl. Serve.

Sweet Chili Garlic Sauce

Just because you need to go garlic-free on the low-FODMAP diet doesn't mean you have to go without one of the best sauces around. Asafetida powder gives this sauce a garlicky taste, and sugar and vinegar give it sweetness and zippy tang. Use this on top of salmon or shrimp, in a stir-fry, as a sauce for a Thai-inspired pizza, or as a dipping sauce for panko-crusted chicken. The sauce can be stored at room temperature for 1 month or in the refrigerator for up to 6 months.

1 pound chili peppers, ends trimmed

1/16 teaspoon wheat-free asafetida powder

2 tablespoons safflower oil

1/4 cup rice wine vinegar

1/4 cup light brown sugar

1/4 cup gluten-free fish sauce

Makes 2½ cups
Per Serving (Serving size: ½ cup)
Calories 116
Fat 5g
Protein 2g
Sodium 1,140mg
Fiber 1g
Carbohydrates 15g
Sugar 12g

1. To a food processor, add chili peppers and asafetida. Process until minced.
2. In a medium sauté pan over medium-high heat, heat oil until shimmering. Add chili pepper mixture, and cook 1 minute. Add vinegar, sugar, and fish sauce, and stir to combine. Reduce heat to low and cook 25 minutes.
3. Use immediately, or pour into an airtight container or canning jar for storage.

Pumpkin Maple Glaze

Don't wait for fall—dazzle your family or guests any time of year by dressing up your carved roast chicken with this fast, delicious autumnal glaze.

Makes ½ cup	
Per Serving **(Serving size: 1 tablespoon)**	
Calories	68
Fat	4g
Protein	1g
Sodium	72mg
Fiber	0g
Carbohydrates	6g
Sugar	5g

¼ cup hulled pumpkin seeds

2 tablespoons unsalted butter, melted, divided

⅛ teaspoon sea salt

3 tablespoons pure maple syrup, divided

1 tablespoon Dijon mustard

1. Preheat broiler. Spread pumpkin seeds on a lined baking sheet. Drizzle 1 tablespoon butter over pumpkin seeds. Sprinkle seeds with salt, and toss to coat. Broil 1–2 minutes or until seeds start to brown lightly.
2. Transfer seeds to a serving dish and mix in 1 tablespoon syrup.
3. In a saucepan over medium heat, combine remaining 1 tablespoon butter, remaining 2 tablespoons syrup, and mustard. Bring just to a boil, then lower heat and simmer, uncovered, 1–2 minutes more to thicken.
4. The glaze and roasted seeds can be used to top any roasted poultry.

Tzatziki Dressing

This smooth dressing can be drizzled over grilled meat or fish or used to liven up a salad. It captures the flavors and nutrients of traditional tzatziki sauce. Even garlic plays a role via infused oil. This dressing can be stored in an airtight container in the refrigerator for up to 2 days.

½ medium cucumber, seeded and diced

½ cup lactose-free plain yogurt

1 teaspoon garlic-infused olive oil

1 tablespoon fresh lemon juice

1 tablespoon chopped dill

Place all ingredients in a blender and process until smooth. Serve.

Makes 1 cup

Per Serving
(Serving size: ¼ cup)

Calories	28
Fat	1g
Protein	1g
Sodium	19mg
Fiber	0g
Carbohydrates	4g
Sugar	2g

Tahini Dressing

This nutty dressing pairs well with Lemon Kale Salad (Chapter 9). This dressing can be stored in an airtight container at room temperature for 1–2 weeks.

¼ cup tahini

¼ cup water

2 tablespoons fresh lemon juice

1 tablespoon pure maple syrup

¼ teaspoon pink Himalayan salt

¼ teaspoon ground black pepper

Combine all ingredients in a blender or food processor. Serve.

Makes ¾ cup

Per Serving
(Serving size: 2 tablespoons)

Calories	66
Fat	5g
Protein	2g
Sodium	72mg
Fiber	1g
Carbohydrates	5g
Sugar	2g

Blueberry Chia Seed Jam

The blueberry flavor sings in this jam. Try it on your favorite breakfast treats or breads or on crackers for a snack. You can also make this jam with ½ pint (6 ounces) of fresh strawberries. This jam can be stored in the refrigerator for 2 weeks or frozen for up to 2 months.

Makes 1 cup
Per Serving
(Serving size: 2 tablespoons)
Calories 37
Fat 1g
Protein 0g
Sodium 1mg
Fiber 1g
Carbohydrates 8g
Sugar 6g

½ pint (6 ounces) blueberries

1 tablespoon lemon juice

2½ tablespoons pure maple syrup

1 tablespoon chia seeds

1. To a small saucepan over medium-high heat, add blueberries, lemon juice, and syrup. Cover. Stir occasionally until fruit breaks down and begins to thicken, about 10 minutes.
2. Uncover and cook mixture at a boil until it develops a sauce-like consistency, about 5 minutes.
3. Stir in chia seeds and cook 2 more minutes. Stir again and then remove from heat.
4. Transfer jam to an airtight jar or other container, and allow to cool or refrigerate 2–3 hours before use. The jam will continue to thicken.

Caesar Salad Dressing

Eating a low-FODMAP diet doesn't mean you have to give up creamy, delicious Caesar salad; you just need to modify it a bit. You can store this dressing in an airtight container in the refrigerator for 3–4 days.

6 anchovy fillets packed in oil, drained and chopped

1/16 teaspoon wheat-free asafetida powder

2 large egg yolks

2 tablespoons fresh lemon juice

3/4 teaspoon Dijon mustard

2 tablespoons garlic-infused olive oil

1/2 cup extra-virgin olive oil

3 tablespoons finely grated Parmesan cheese

1/4 teaspoon kosher salt

1 teaspoon ground black pepper

Makes 1 cup	
Per Serving **(Serving size: 2 tablespoons)**	
Calories	179
Fat	18g
Protein	2g
Sodium	217mg
Fiber	0g
Carbohydrates	1g
Sugar	0g

1. In a small bowl, use a fork to mash anchovies and asafetida into a paste, then place in a medium bowl.
2. Whisk in egg yolks, lemon juice, and mustard. Slowly whisk in garlic-infused oil and then olive oil.
3. Whisk in Parmesan, salt, and pepper. Serve.

Ginger Sesame Salad Dressing

Spruce up tofu or chicken with this dressing, or use it for an Asian-inspired salad or to top vegetables in collard green wraps. This dressing can be stored for 1 week in the refrigerator.

Makes 1 cup

Per Serving
(Serving size: 2 tablespoons)

Calories 139
Fat 14g
Protein 0g
Sodium 251mg
Fiber 0g
Carbohydrates 3g
Sugar 3g

Ginger for Health

Ginger has long been prized for its health benefits. It's said to soothe nausea, support the immune system, and have strong anti-inflammatory effects. Fresh ginger can be stored in your refrigerator for up to 3 weeks or in the freezer for up to 6 months.

½ cup extra-virgin olive oil

¼ cup rice wine vinegar

2 tablespoons gluten-free soy sauce (tamari)

2 tablespoons demerara sugar

1 teaspoon sesame oil

1 (1-inch) piece ginger, peeled and minced

In a blender or food processor, blend all ingredients until smooth. Serve immediately, or put in a container for storage. If dressing is chilled, bring to room temperature before serving.

Thai Peanut Dressing

Use this dressing in Collard Green Wraps with Thai Peanut Dressing (see recipe in Chapter 7), or add it to salads, other wraps, or sandwiches. You can store this dressing in an airtight container in the refrigerator for up to 3 days.

¼ cup creamy natural peanut butter

2 tablespoons rice wine vinegar

Juice of 1 medium lime

1 tablespoon gluten-free soy sauce (tamari)

2 tablespoons pure maple syrup

2½ tablespoons light brown sugar

¹⁄₁₆ teaspoon wheat-free asafetida powder

1½ tablespoons peeled, grated ginger

1 teaspoon Himalayan salt

¼ teaspoon chili powder

Makes ¾ cup	
Per Serving (Serving size: 2 tablespoons)	
Calories	99
Fat	5g
Protein	3g
Sodium	434mg
Fiber	1g
Carbohydrates	11g
Sugar	9g

Place all ingredients in a food processor and pulse until combined. Serve.

Pomegranate Salsa

Use this beautiful and tasty salsa on fish or poultry, or scoop it up with tortilla chips.

Makes 4 cups

Per Serving
(Serving size: ¼ cup)

Calories	32
Fat	0g
Protein	1g
Sodium	13mg
Fiber	1g
Carbohydrates	7g
Sugar	5g

Remember Your Low-FODMAP Servings

Dipping into salsa or dips can be fun, but you still need to mind how many servings of certain foods you consume. Enjoy this salsa, but do your best to only have ¼ cup.

1⅓ cups diced cucumber

2½ cups pomegranate seeds

⅓ cup finely chopped cilantro

Juice of ½ medium lime

1 tablespoon pure maple syrup

2 tablespoons slivered almonds

⅛ teaspoon sea salt

1. To a medium bowl, add cucumber and pomegranate.
2. In a small bowl, place cilantro, lime juice, syrup, almonds, and salt, and stir to combine.
3. Add contents of small bowl to cucumber and pomegranate, and toss gently to combine. Serve.

Fiesta Salsa

Use this salsa as a dip for tortilla chips or nachos, mix it with mayonnaise for a bold kick, or stir it into scrambled eggs. You can store this salsa in an airtight container in the refrigerator for 5–7 days.

1 (10-ounce) can diced tomatoes, drained

1 (14.5-ounce) can diced tomatoes with green chilies

1 tablespoon garlic-infused olive oil

¼ cup chopped green onions, green parts only

¼ cup chopped cilantro

¼ cup chopped flat-leaf parsley

⅛ teaspoon wheat-free asafetida powder

¼ teaspoon ground cumin

¼ teaspoon coriander

¼ teaspoon dried oregano

¼ teaspoon smoked paprika

¼ teaspoon sea salt

½ teaspoon ground black pepper

Juice of 1 medium lime

Add all ingredients to a medium serving bowl. Stir well to combine. Serve.

Serves 6

Per Serving

Calories	49
Fat	2g
Protein	1g
Sodium	361mg
Fiber	2g
Carbohydrates	6g
Sugar	3g

Tomato Tip!

When shopping for canned tomatoes, especially those made with chilies, make sure the ingredients do not include high-FODMAP ingredients such as onions, garlic, onion powder, or garlic powder.

CHAPTER 11

Desserts

Mixed Berry Cobbler

Moist and slightly sweet, this dessert is perfect to make in summer when fresh berries are abundant. Rustic, comforting, and delicious, this dessert is sure to delight you and your guests.

Serves 8

Per Serving

Calories 305
Fat 13g
Protein 4g
Sodium 193mg
Fiber 4g
Carbohydrates 41g
Sugar 14g

2 teaspoons ground cinnamon, divided

1 cup gluten-free all-purpose flour

½ teaspoon xanthan gum

3 tablespoons granulated sugar

1½ teaspoons gluten-free baking powder

¼ teaspoon salt

1 large egg

1 cup lactose-free milk

3 cups mixed blueberries, raspberries, and sliced strawberries

Zest of ½ large lemon

1 cup quick-cooking oats

¼ cup (firmly packed) light brown sugar

8 tablespoons unsalted butter, softened

1. Preheat oven to 400°F. Grease an 8" × 8" baking dish.
2. Using a stand mixer on low speed, mix together 1 teaspoon cinnamon, flour, xanthan gum, sugar, baking powder, and salt. Add egg and milk, and mix on medium speed until well combined.
3. Pour into prepared baking dish. Top with mixed fruit and lemon zest.
4. In the stand mixer on low speed, combine oats, brown sugar, butter, and remaining 1 teaspoon cinnamon. Crumble mixture on top of fruit.
5. Bake 35 minutes. Serve.

Pumpkin Spice Cupcakes with Buttercream Frosting

When autumn magic is in the air, take advantage and make this heartwarming treat. Remember to chill this low-lactose frosting and let the cupcakes cool completely before you bring the two together.

Cupcakes

½ cup unsalted butter at room temperature

½ cup turbinado sugar

¼ cup (firmly packed) light brown sugar

½ cup canned pumpkin

1 large egg

½ teaspoon alcohol-free vanilla extract

1¼ cups gluten-free all-purpose flour

½ teaspoon baking soda

½ teaspoon gluten-free baking powder

1 teaspoon ground cinnamon

¼ teaspoon Himalayan sea salt

Frosting

½ cup dairy-free margarine

2 cups confectioners' sugar

½ teaspoon alcohol-free vanilla extract

1 tablespoon unsweetened almond milk

½ tablespoon lactose-free plain yogurt

Makes 12 cupcakes, 1¼ cups frosting

Per Serving (Serving size: 1 cupcake)

Calories	322
Fat	15g
Protein	1g
Sodium	176mg
Fiber	0g
Carbohydrates	44g
Sugar	30g

1. Preheat oven to 350°F.
2. For the cupcakes, using a stand mixer, cream together butter and sugars on medium speed until fluffy. Add pumpkin, egg, and vanilla extract, and mix until blended.
3. In a medium bowl, stir together flour, baking soda, baking powder, cinnamon, and salt. Add to mixer bowl, and mix on low speed.
4. Fill cups of an ungreased nonstick muffin pan ⅔ full with batter. Bake 12 minutes or until a toothpick inserted into the center of a cupcake comes out clean. Remove cupcakes from pan, and transfer to racks to cool.
5. For frosting, using a stand mixer or an electric hand mixer with a large mixing bowl, cream margarine at low speed, and gradually add confectioners' sugar, mixing until combined.
6. Set speed to high, add remaining frosting ingredients, and beat until smooth and creamy. Be sure to chill 30–60 minutes in refrigerator before using on cupcakes.

Maple Cinnamon Coconut Chia Seed Pudding

This is a delicious dessert that could also be enjoyed for breakfast. Filled with fruit, nuts, and chia seeds and the sweetness of maple syrup, this pudding will fulfill your sugar cravings and keep you feeling full and satisfied.

Serves 4

Per Serving

Calories	239
Fat	11g
Protein	5g
Sodium	49mg
Fiber	9g
Carbohydrates	33g
Sugar	17g

Chia Seed Pudding Options

Try replacing the almond milk in your chia seed pudding with milk made from coconut, hemp, or soy. Add low-FODMAP spices such as pumpkin spice, curry, or nutmeg. Or experiment with toppings: Use your favorite low-FODMAP fruits, and choose low-FODMAP nuts such as almonds, hazelnuts, macadamia nuts, Brazil nuts, or pecans.

¼ cup chia seeds

1 cup unsweetened almond milk

2 tablespoons pure maple syrup

½ teaspoon alcohol-free vanilla extract

½ teaspoon ground cinnamon

2 tablespoons shredded unsweetened coconut

2 medium bananas, sliced

20 medium strawberries, chopped

¼ cup chopped walnuts

1. In a large bowl, mix chia seeds, almond milk, syrup, vanilla, cinnamon, and coconut. Allow to sit at room temperature 40 minutes to 1 hour, stirring every 10–15 minutes, then cover with plastic wrap and refrigerate overnight.
2. In four ice cream glasses, canning jars, or bowls, layer bananas, pudding, and strawberries. Top with walnuts. Serve.

Blueberry Granola Crisp

Moist, lightly sweet, and berry delicious! Bring this crisp to a barbecue or a winter holiday party, or share it for dessert after brunch. Try it with lactose-free, wheat-free ice cream.

3 cups blueberries

1 tablespoon cornstarch

2½ cups rolled oats

⅔ cup melted coconut oil

1 cup brown rice flour

⅓ cup turbinado sugar

¼ cup chopped macadamia nuts

¼ cup chopped walnuts

1 teaspoon ground cinnamon

½ teaspoon ground ginger

¼ teaspoon ground nutmeg

Serves 8	
Per Serving	
Calories	445
Fat	25g
Protein	6g
Sodium	2mg
Fiber	6g
Carbohydrates	51g
Sugar	15g

1. Preheat oven to 350°F.
2. In a 9" × 13" baking dish, combine blueberries and cornstarch. Mix well. Set aside.
3. In a large bowl, mix together remaining ingredients until well combined. Spread mixture evenly over blueberries.
4. Bake 50–60 minutes or until top starts to brown. Serve warm.

Peanut Butter Chocolate Mug Cake

When you have a craving for peanut butter and chocolate, try this recipe and feed your craving in a low-FODMAP way in under 5 minutes.

Serves 1

Per Serving

Calories 408
Fat 21g
Protein 8g
Sodium 150mg
Fiber 3g
Carbohydrates 46g
Sugar 22g

2 tablespoons gluten-free all-purpose flour

2 tablespoons unsweetened almond milk

1 tablespoon pure maple syrup

2 tablespoons creamy natural peanut butter

¼ teaspoon gluten-free baking powder

¼ teaspoon ground nutmeg

¼ teaspoon ground cinnamon

½ teaspoon alcohol-free vanilla extract

1 tablespoon dark chocolate chips

1. Add all ingredients except chocolate chips to a microwave-safe mug, and stir well until combined.
2. Microwave mug 1–2 minutes. Microwave ovens vary, so check every 30 seconds. Once cake rises, your mug cake is ready. Top with chocolate chips. Serve.

Nut-Free Cranberry Granola Bars

These bars are great for school lunches and, of course, for anyone with a nut allergy. Make batches ahead of time to bring to school or work or to carry as a gut-friendly snack while out and about.

2 cups oats

½ cup puffed rice cereal

½ cup plus 2 teaspoons oat flour

2 tablespoons light brown sugar

½ teaspoon Himalayan sea salt

¼ cup flaxseed meal

3 tablespoons coconut oil

½ cup plus 1 tablespoon pure maple syrup

½ cup no-sugar-added dried cranberries

2 tablespoons dark chocolate chips

Makes 2 dozen bars	
Per Serving (Serving size: 1 bar)	
Calories	84
Fat	3g
Protein	2g
Sodium	34mg
Fiber	1g
Carbohydrates	13g
Sugar	5g

1. Preheat oven to 350°F. Line a 9" × 13" baking pan with parchment paper.
2. To the bowl of a stand mixer, add oats, cereal, oat flour, sugar, salt, and flaxseed, and mix on low speed to combine.
3. In a small bowl, combine oil, syrup, cranberries, and chocolate chips. Add to mixer and mix on low speed with other ingredients until combined.
4. Use a spatula to spread mixture out evenly in prepared pan.
5. Place another piece of parchment paper on top of mixture and use a heavy, flat object (such as a cutting board) to press down evenly and firmly to flatten. Remove parchment paper and bake 16–18 minutes (don't throw top layer of parchment paper away).
6. Once done baking, use parchment paper and heavy object to flatten bars again.
7. Place pan on top of a baking sheet, and refrigerate 20 minutes. This will give bars a slightly chewier texture and make them easier to cut. (Leaving pan to cool at room temperature before cutting is not recommended.) Cut into 24 bars and serve.

Peanut Butter Cookies

With a short ingredients list that's long on flavor, these cookies are easy and quick to make. Bake them for the kids in your life, for bake sales or potlucks, or just to enjoy as a sweet treat.

Makes 18 cookies
Per Serving
(Serving size: 1 cookie)
Calories 137
Fat 7g
Protein 4g
Sodium 28mg
Fiber 1g
Carbohydrates 15g
Sugar 13g

1 cup natural peanut butter

1 cup turbinado sugar

1 teaspoon alcohol-free vanilla extract

1 tablespoon pure maple syrup

1 large egg

¼ teaspoon coarse Himalayan sea salt

1. Preheat oven to 350°F.
2. In a medium bowl, mix together peanut butter, sugar, vanilla, syrup, and egg.
3. Spoon about 1 tablespoon dough for each cookie, and place balls about 1 inch apart on an ungreased baking sheet. Use the prongs of a fork to gently press down and flatten each cookie. Turn fork and press down again to make a crosshatch pattern. Lightly sprinkle salt on top of cookies.
4. Bake 5 minutes, then turn baking sheet 180 degrees and continue baking 5 more minutes or until golden brown around the edges. Let cool and serve.

Chocolate Chip Cookies

Chocolate chip cookies just taste like childhood. Warm and gooey, these chocolaty delights will fulfill your nostalgia and sugar cravings without all the gut-disturbing ingredients of store-bought cookies.

2 cups gluten-free all-purpose flour

1 cup (lightly packed) light brown sugar

1 teaspoon baking soda

1 teaspoon gluten-free baking powder

½ teaspoon Himalayan salt

½ cup safflower oil

1 tablespoon pure maple syrup

¼ cup unsweetened almond milk

1¼ tablespoons alcohol-free vanilla extract

1 cup dark chocolate chips

Makes 24 cookies	
Per Serving (Serving size: 1 cookie)	
Calories	181
Fat	8g
Protein	1g
Sodium	109mg
Fiber	1g
Carbohydrates	26g
Sugar	13g

1. Preheat oven to 350°F.
2. In a large bowl, combine flour, sugar, baking soda, baking powder, and salt.
3. To the bowl of a stand mixer, add oil, syrup, almond milk, and vanilla, and mix on medium speed.
4. Add dry ingredients, and mix on low speed until smooth. Gradually add chocolate chips.
5. Drop rounded tablespoons of dough onto a nonstick baking sheet. This mixture will be slightly wet.
6. Bake cookies 12–14 minutes until lightly brown. Longer baking yields crispier cookies.

Peppermint Patties

Made with coconut milk and unsweetened coconut, these sweet, fun candies are perfect to drop in a lunch bag or to indulge in as a low-FODMAP after-dinner treat. Store any leftovers in an airtight container in the refrigerator for up to 2 weeks, or in the freezer for up to 2 months.

Makes 24 patties

Per Serving
(Serving size: 1 patty)

Calories	192
Fat	13g
Protein	1g
Sodium	1mg
Fiber	3g
Carbohydrates	17g
Sugar	12g

2 cups shredded unsweetened coconut

¼ cup coconut milk

¼ cup coconut oil

½ cup pure maple syrup

½ teaspoon alcohol-free peppermint extract

2 cups dark chocolate chips

1. In a food processor, process shredded coconut until it reaches a fine texture, about 30 seconds. Add coconut milk, oil, syrup, and peppermint extract, and pulse to make a paste.
2. Shape paste into 1½-inch rounds, and place on a baking sheet lined with parchment paper. Place rounds in freezer 10 minutes.
3. Place 1 inch water in a medium skillet over a burner. Place chocolate chips in a heatproof glass bowl, and place bowl directly in water. Bring water to a simmer, then turn off heat and let chocolate sit until melted. Stir.
4. Remove patties from freezer. Place a patty on tines of a fork, and dip into melted chocolate to completely cover. Return patty to parchment paper–lined baking sheet, and repeat with all patties.
5. Allow chocolate shells to cool and harden before serving.

Nutty Fudge

Here's a creamy, chocolaty delicacy. This recipe uses coconut milk and maple syrup to obtain the smooth texture that makes fudge a delight. Store this treat between pieces of waxed paper at room temperature in an airtight container for 1–2 weeks, in the refrigerator for 2–3 weeks, or in the freezer for 3 months if properly wrapped.

1 (13.5-ounce) can coconut milk

¼ cup pure maple syrup

1¾ cups dark chocolate chips

⅛ teaspoon Himalayan salt

½ tablespoon alcohol-free vanilla extract

½ cup chopped walnuts

Makes 64 squares
Per Serving **(Serving size: 1 square)**
Calories 56
Fat 4g
Protein 0g
Sodium 3mg
Fiber 1g
Carbohydrates 5g
Sugar 3g

1. Line an 8" × 8" baking pan with parchment paper. Set aside.
2. In a medium saucepan over medium-high heat, bring coconut milk to a boil. Reduce heat to low, and simmer 5 minutes, stirring occasionally.
3. Whisk in syrup, and simmer 25 more minutes.
4. Remove from heat. Stir in chocolate chips, salt, and vanilla, and continue stirring until chocolate is melted. Stir in nuts. Pour mixture into prepared pan.
5. Refrigerate at least 2 hours or until set. Cut into 1-inch squares. Serve.

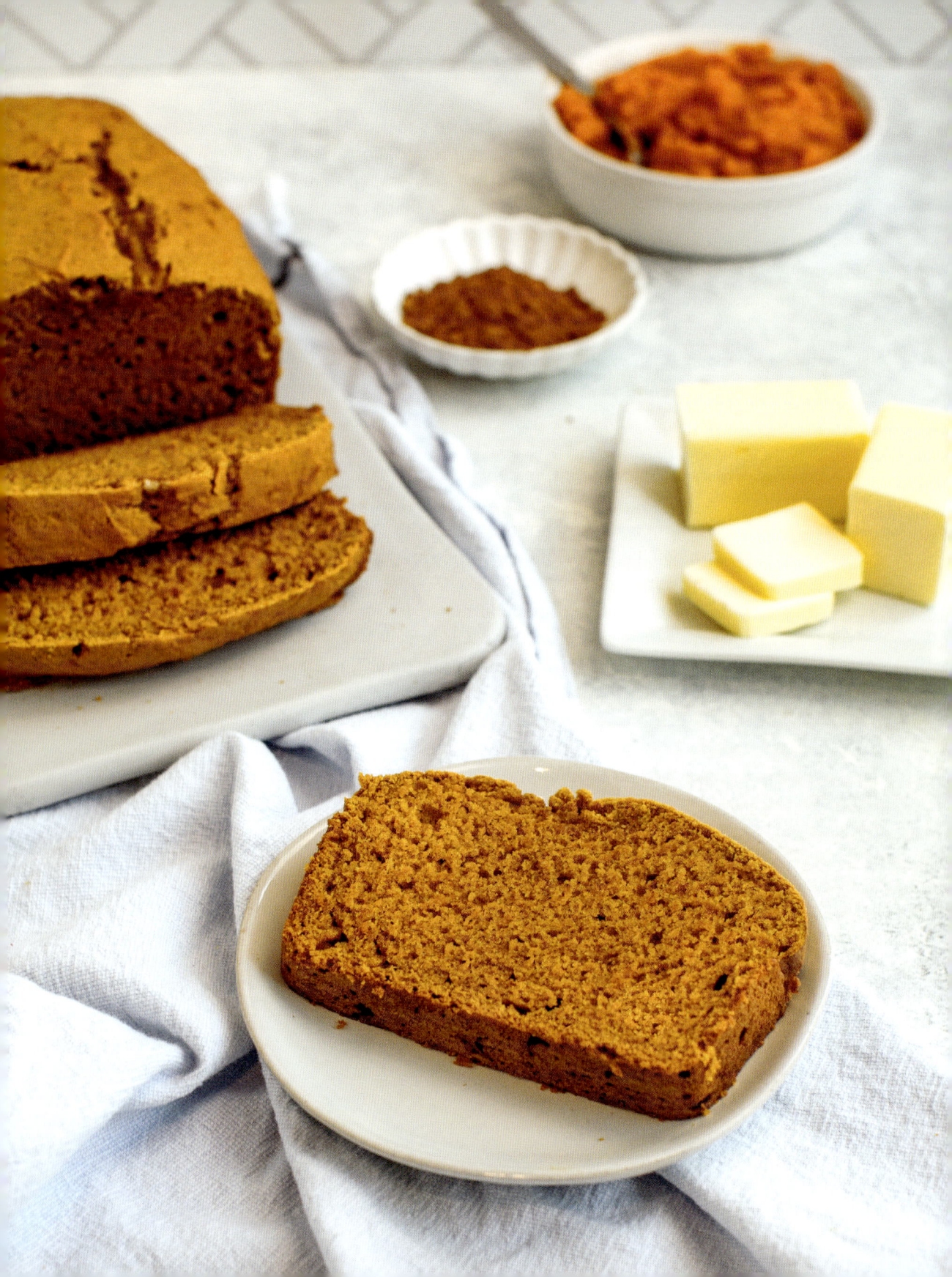

Pumpkin Bread

Perfect for the holidays or a cold weekend, warm pumpkin bread from the oven is so heavenly!

½ cup unsalted butter

1 cup sugar

2 large eggs

1 teaspoon alcohol-free vanilla extract

1 (15-ounce) can pumpkin purée

2 cups gluten-free all-purpose flour

1 tablespoon orange zest

½ tablespoon ground cinnamon

1½ teaspoons pumpkin pie spice

1 teaspoon baking soda

½ teaspoon salt

Serves 8	
Per Serving	
Calories	388
Fat	12g
Protein	4g
Sodium	324mg
Fiber	2g
Carbohydrates	62g
Sugar	27g

1. Preheat oven to 325°F. Lightly grease a 9" × 5" loaf pan.
2. Using a stand mixer, cream butter and sugar on medium speed until light and fluffy. Add eggs one at a time, mixing well after each. Add vanilla and pumpkin and mix until well blended.
3. In a separate large bowl, mix together flour, orange zest, cinnamon, pumpkin pie spice, baking soda, and salt. Gradually add flour mixture to pumpkin mixture, and mix until combined. Do not overmix.
4. Pour into prepared pan and bake 60–70 minutes or until a toothpick inserted into the center comes out clean. Serve.

Molasses Cookies

Sweet, dark, and spicy, these warming cookies are perfect to bake when the weather starts to cool. Sorghum flour is a gluten-free flour with a mild flavor and smooth texture—perfect for baking cookies like these.

Makes 18 cookies
Per Serving (Serving size: 1 cookie)
Calories 93
Fat 1g
Protein 1g
Sodium 41mg
Fiber 0g
Carbohydrates 20g
Sugar 13g

¾ cup plus 2 tablespoons sorghum flour

½ teaspoon baking soda

1 teaspoon ground cinnamon

1 teaspoon ground ginger

1½ tablespoons unsalted butter, softened

½ cup (packed) dark brown sugar

1 large egg

2 tablespoons molasses

½ cup turbinado sugar

1. Preheat oven to 375°F. Spray a large baking sheet with cooking spray.
2. To the bowl of a stand mixer, add flour, baking soda, cinnamon, and ginger. Mix on low speed to combine, and set aside.
3. In a large bowl, whisk together butter and brown sugar until fluffy. Add egg, and beat to incorporate. Add molasses and mix until well combined. Add to bowl with dry ingredients. Mix on medium speed until combined.
4. Place turbinado sugar on a small, shallow plate. Scoop out 1½–2 tablespoons dough, roll into a ball, and then flatten into a disk between your hands. Dip dough disk into turbinado sugar, pressing gently if needed to get sugar to stick. Repeat with all dough, placing sugared disks on prepared baking sheet 1–2 inches apart.
5. Bake cookies 8 minutes. Cookies should have a gooey texture. Cool on a rack and serve.

Chai Spice Cookies

These are the perfect chewy cookies for the fall and winter holidays. They have a little bit of sweetness and a little bit of spice. Make them as a low-FODMAP contribution to a cookie swap or as a dessert for yourself at home.

¾ cup plus 2 tablespoons (lightly packed) light brown sugar

1¼ teaspoons ground cinnamon

½ teaspoon ground cardamom

½ teaspoon ground ginger

¼ teaspoon ground allspice

⅛ teaspoon ground black pepper

⅛ teaspoon ground cloves

½ cup unsalted butter at room temperature

1¼ cups gluten-free all-purpose flour

¼ teaspoon gluten-free baking powder

½ teaspoon baking soda

¼ teaspoon Himalayan salt

1 large egg at room temperature

½ teaspoon alcohol-free vanilla extract

Makes 15 cookies

Per Serving
(Serving size: 1 cookie)

Calories 157
Fat 6g
Protein 1g
Sodium 85mg
Fiber 0g
Carbohydrates 24g
Sugar 12g

Gluten-Free Flours

While regular all-purpose flour is made of just one grain (wheat), gluten-free all-purpose flour consists of a blend of several. You can try various brands of store-bought all-purpose gluten-free flour (each uses its own combination of grains) or make your own using one of the recipes in Chapter 2.

---

1. Preheat oven to 350°F. Line a baking sheet with parchment paper.
2. In the bowl of a stand mixer on low speed, combine sugar, cinnamon, cardamom, ginger, allspice, pepper, and cloves. Remove 2 tablespoons of sugar–spice mixture and set aside on a wide plate or rimmed baking sheet. Fit mixer with a paddle attachment, add butter, and beat on medium speed until fluffy, about 2 minutes.
3. In a large bowl, sift together flour, baking powder, baking soda, and salt, and set aside.
4. Add egg and vanilla to butter mixture, and beat until fully incorporated. Slowly add flour mixture, and mix until combined.
5. Roll dough between palms into 1-inch balls. Roll each ball in reserved spice mixture, and place on prepared baking sheet about 1 inch apart.
6. Bake 8–10 minutes. Cookies should be golden and slightly puffed, with a cracked surface. Let stand on baking sheet 2–3 minutes before transferring to wire racks to cool. Serve.

Coconut Balls

Sweet and crunchy, these charming confections are pretty as can be. If you're feeling fancy, give them a fine drizzle of melted dark chocolate, or lightly sprinkle them with cinnamon or confectioners' sugar.

Makes 15 cookies

Per Serving
(Serving size: 1 cookie)

Calories 113
Fat 9g
Protein 1g
Sodium 20mg
Fiber 2g
Carbohydrates 8g
Sugar 5g

2 cups shredded unsweetened coconut

2½ tablespoons melted coconut oil

2 tablespoons rice flour

2 large egg whites (about ⅓ cup)

¼ cup cane sugar

1 teaspoon alcohol-free vanilla extract

⅛ teaspoon sea salt

½ tablespoon pure maple syrup

1. Preheat oven to 350°F.
2. In the bowl of a stand mixer, combine coconut, oil, and flour on low speed.
3. In a small bowl, whisk together egg whites, sugar, vanilla, and salt. Add to flour mixture, and mix on medium speed 30–45 seconds. Add syrup, and mix until fully combined.
4. Gently shape mixture into 1-inch balls and place on a nonstick baking sheet.
5. Bake 15–20 minutes until firm but tender. Remove from oven and let stand 30–60 minutes. Consuming right away may cause coconut balls to crumble.

CHAPTER 12

Drinks

Warm Ginger Tea

When your gut is having a bad day, sit down with this cup of tea. Sip slowly and relax.

Serves 1

Per Serving

Calories 21
Fat 0g
Protein 0g
Sodium 390mg
Fiber 0g
Carbohydrates 6g
Sugar 4g

1 cup boiling water

1 (2-inch) piece ginger, peeled and grated

Juice of ½ medium lemon

1 teaspoon pure maple syrup

¼ teaspoon ground black pepper

¼ teaspoon Himalayan salt

Pour water into a teacup, and add all ingredients. Let sit 2–3 minutes. Serve.

Ginger Maple Tea

Soothe your tummy with the best comforts of ginger, lemon, cinnamon, and maple syrup.

Serves 1

Per Serving

Calories 60
Fat 0g
Protein 0g
Sodium 2mg
Fiber 1g
Carbohydrates 16g
Sugar 12g

1 cup boiling water, divided

1 teaspoon peeled, grated ginger

2 slices lemon

1 teaspoon ground cinnamon

1 tablespoon pure maple syrup

1. Pour ¾ cup water into mug. Add ginger, lemon, cinnamon, and syrup, and allow to steep 10 minutes.
2. Add remaining ¼ cup water. Serve and sip slowly.

Carrot Pineapple Ginger Juice

When you need some help getting your digestive tract moving, this juice is refreshing and delightful for the tummy.

2 cups pineapple chunks

1 large carrot, peeled and chopped

3 tablespoons peeled, grated ginger

½ teaspoon cayenne pepper

Add all ingredients to a juicer or food processor. Blend well, and strain through a sieve. Serve in glasses.

Serves 2	
Per Serving	
Calories	53
Fat	0g
Protein	0g
Sodium	6mg
Fiber	0g
Carbohydrates	13g
Sugar	10g

Cucumber Melon Water

When you're tired of plain water, this refreshing drink will leave you cool as a cucumber!

Serves 2	
Per Serving	
Calories	3
Fat	0g
Protein	0g
Sodium	0mg
Fiber	0g
Carbohydrates	1g
Sugar	1g

2½ cups cold water with ice

½ cup sliced cucumber

½ cup cubed honeydew melon

Juice of ½ medium lime

4 mint leaves

Mix together all ingredients in a small pitcher and refrigerate 3–4 hours. Serve.

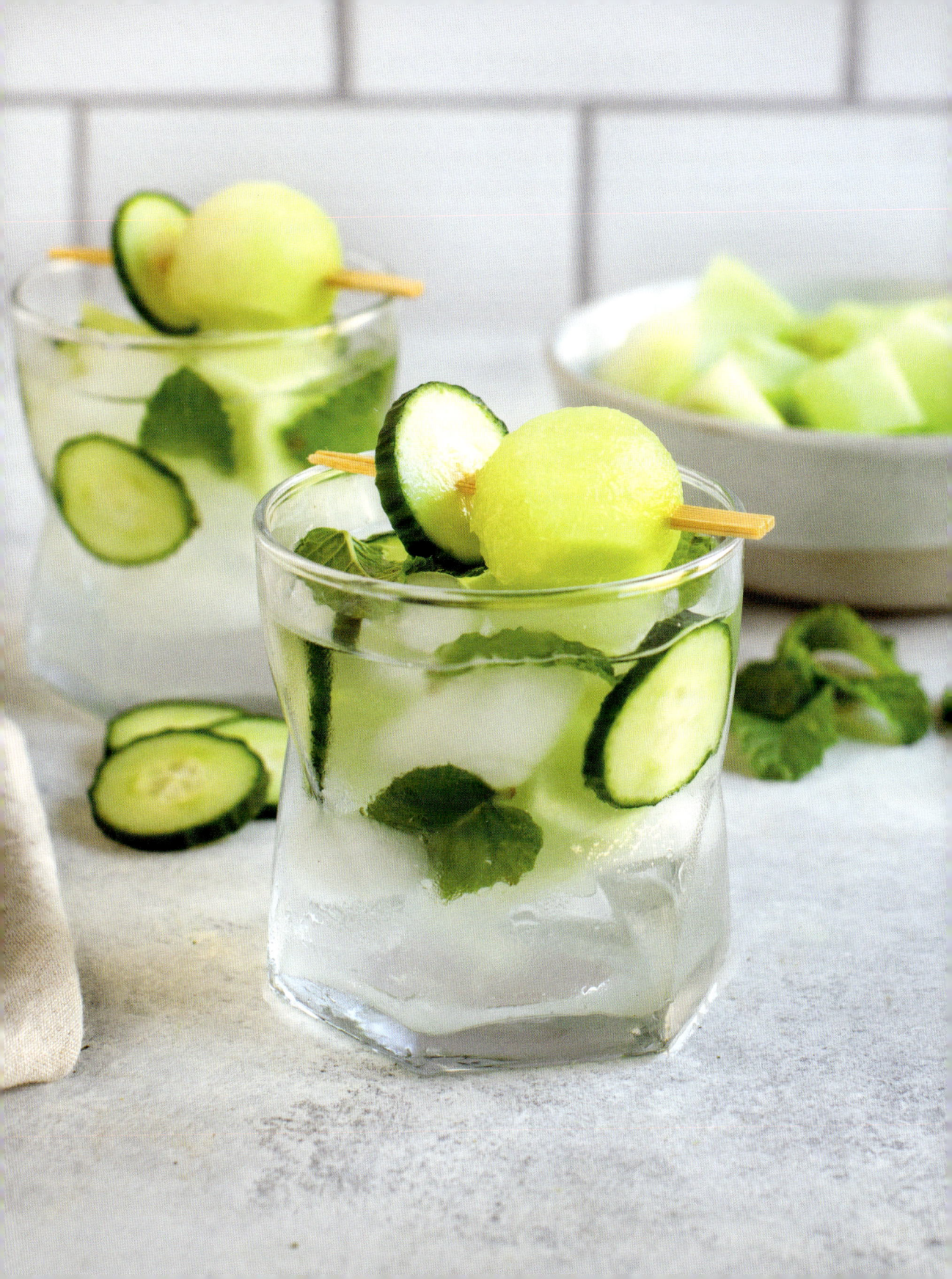

Gut-Friendly Smoothie

Per recent studies, turmeric extract may help reduce IBS symptoms. The curcumin content in turmeric may help with inflammation. This smoothie was created especially for those suffering from IBS.

Serves 1	
Per Serving	
Calories	689
Fat	62g
Protein	8g
Sodium	31mg
Fiber	7g
Carbohydrates	28g
Sugar	7g

1 cup coconut milk

1 tablespoon coconut oil

1 tablespoon chia seeds

½ medium ripe banana

½ teaspoon ground turmeric

½ teaspoon ground cinnamon

Blend all ingredients thoroughly in a blender, and enjoy immediately.

Strawberry Coconut Almond Smoothie

This low-FODMAP smoothie is great for breakfast or lunch, or after a workout.

½ cup ice cubes

½ cup hulled, chopped strawberries

½ cup unsweetened almond milk

¼ cup shredded unsweetened coconut

1 tablespoon smooth almond butter

1 scoop protein powder

Serves 1	
Per Serving	
Calories	375
Fat	22g
Protein	32g
Sodium	328mg
Fiber	8g
Carbohydrates	16g
Sugar	6g

Place all ingredients in a blender and blend until smooth. Serve.

Revival Smoothie

When you need a gut-friendly drink that's filling and quick to make, or if you want a post-workout meal, this smoothie is it.

2 cups spinach

10 frozen blueberries

½ medium ripe banana, frozen

1 tablespoon chia seeds

½ tablespoon hemp seeds

1 scoop protein powder

½ cup water

1 teaspoon unsweetened cocoa powder

Serves 1	
Per Serving	
Calories	275
Fat	7g
Protein	33g
Sodium	286mg
Fiber	9g
Carbohydrates	25g
Sugar	9g

Place all ingredients in a blender and blend until combined. Serve.

Blueberry Ginger Water

This refreshing drink will complement a day in the shade, and it's great when you want some flavor in your fluids.

Makes 1 cup syrup
Per Serving **(Serving size:** **1 tablespoon syrup, plus** **accompaniments)**
Calories 71
Fat 0g
Protein 0g
Sodium 0mg
Fiber 1g
Carbohydrates 18g
Sugar 16g

1 cup coarsely chopped ginger (not peeled)

1 cup turbinado sugar

3 cups water

1 tablespoon lime juice (per serving)

¼ cup blueberries (per serving)

1. Place ginger in a food processor and process until rough in texture.
2. Place ginger, sugar, and water in a medium saucepan. Bring to a boil over high heat, then reduce heat to low and simmer 1 hour, or until liquid is glossy and reduced to 1 cup.
3. Place a sieve over a medium bowl. Strain syrup through sieve, pushing gently down on ginger. Allow syrup to cool slightly, then chill thoroughly in a glass bottle or jar.
4. To use syrup, measure 1 tablespoon into an 8-ounce glass. Add lime juice and blueberries, then fill glass with water and ice. Serve. Store syrup, refrigerated, up to 3 weeks.

Paixão Smoothie

This smoothie is dedicated to the passion fruit and the warm, colorful beaches of Brazil. It's a perfect tropical smoothie for any occasion.

½ medium passion fruit

½ medium ripe banana

1 (6-ounce) tub lactose-free vanilla yogurt

1½ cups unsweetened coconut milk

1 tablespoon coconut cream

1 tablespoon pure maple syrup

1½ cups crushed ice

Serves 2	
Per Serving	
Calories	464
Fat	37g
Protein	8g
Sodium	69mg
Fiber	1g
Carbohydrates	27g
Sugar	18g

Scoop passion fruit pulp and seeds from rind and place in blender with remaining ingredients. Blend until smooth. Pour into two glasses and serve.

Banana Nut Smoothie

This smoothie is great for breakfast. Walnuts are a good source of magnesium, vitamin B_6, and calcium. Garnish with a ripe, red strawberry for a colorful presentation.

½ cup unsweetened soy milk

½ medium ripe banana, frozen

5 frozen strawberries

10 walnut halves

1 cup crushed ice

Serves 1	
Per Serving	
Calories	240
Fat	15g
Protein	8g
Sodium	44mg
Fiber	5g
Carbohydrates	23g
Sugar	11g

Place milk in blender, followed by other ingredients. Blend until smooth and serve.

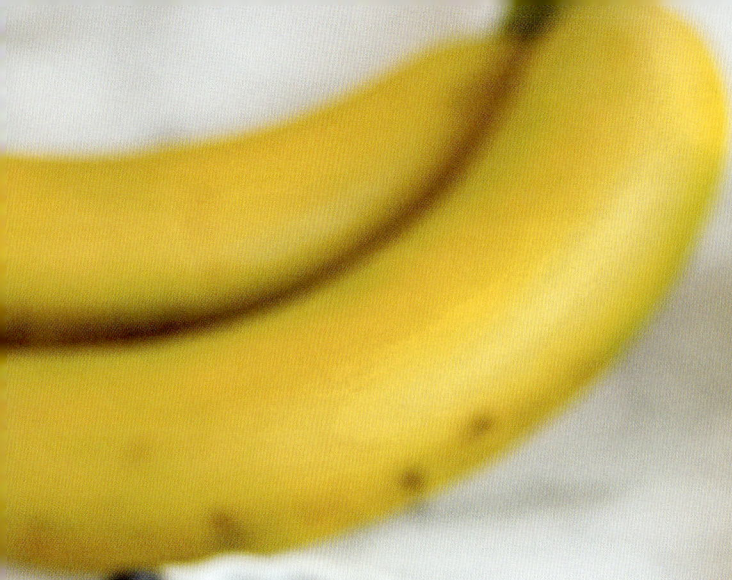

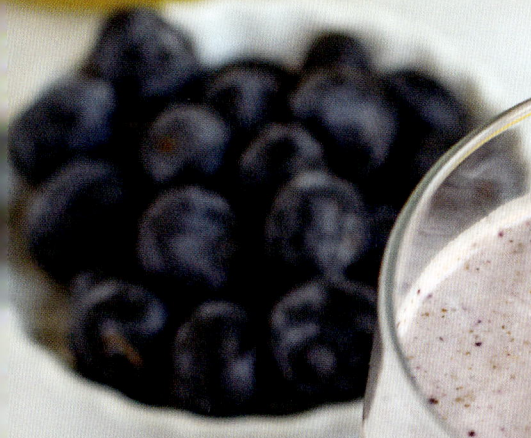

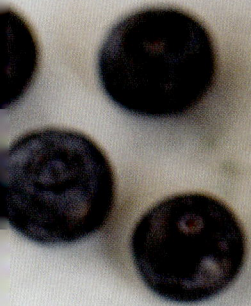

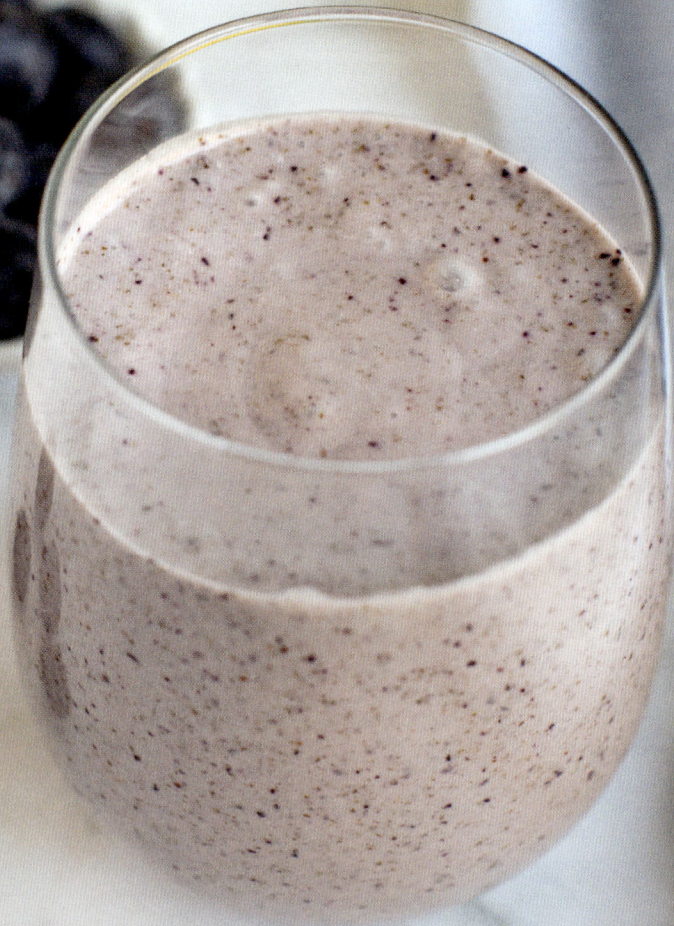

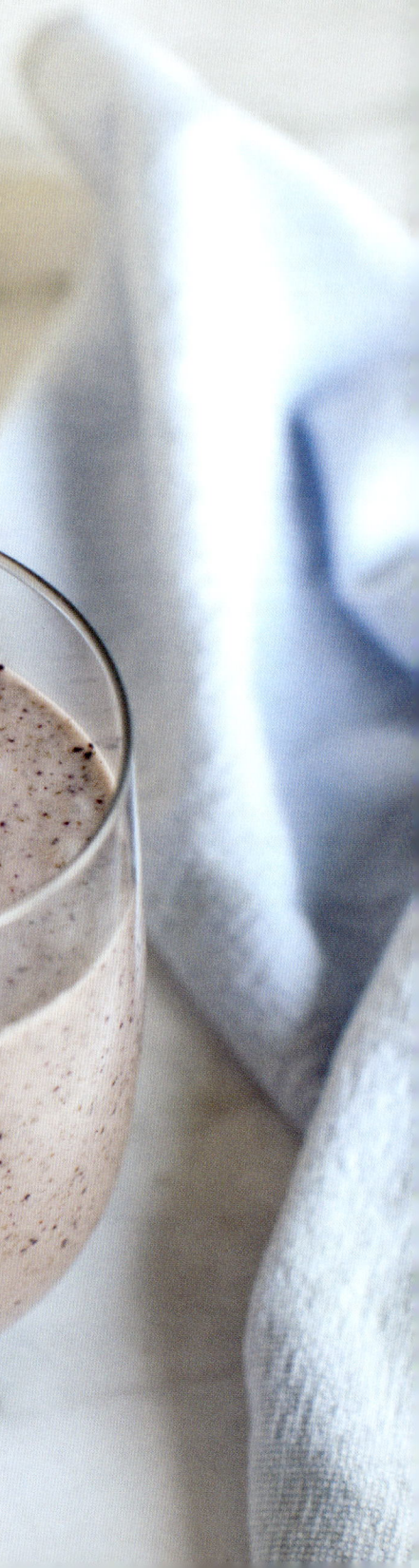

Blue Moon Smoothie

For those who love blueberries and chia seeds, this smoothie is a perfect fit.
If after blending, the mixture is too thin, add more ice.

½ cup unsweetened coconut milk

10 frozen blueberries

½ medium ripe banana

1 tablespoon chia seeds

1 cup crushed ice

Place milk in blender, followed by other ingredients, and
blend until smooth. Serve.

Serves 1	
Per Serving	
Calories	349
Fat	27g
Protein	5g
Sodium	16mg
Fiber	7g
Carbohydrates	25g
Sugar	9g

Peanut Butter–Lover Smoothie

Yummy peanut butter, banana, and avocado make for a creamy and awesome smoothie. If peanut butter is not your thing, you can make this with another low-FODMAP nut butter. If after blending, the mixture is too thick for your taste, add more milk; if it's too thin, add more ice.

Serves 1	
Per Serving	
Calories	690
Fat	56g
Protein	16g
Sodium	84mg
Fiber	4g
Carbohydrates	36g
Sugar	15g

¾ cup unsweetened coconut milk

½ medium ripe banana, frozen

⅛ medium avocado, peeled and pitted

2 tablespoons peanut butter

½ cup lactose-free plain yogurt

½ cup crushed ice

Place milk in blender, followed by other ingredients, and blend until smooth. Serve.

Shamrock Shake

Creamy and minty, this shake is sure to brighten your day—and, with healthy avocado and lettuce, this green treat is a better option for your gut than the processed sugar-packed shakes from fast food joints. You could also use a handful of baby spinach in place of the lettuce if you'd prefer. If after blending, the mixture is too thick for your taste, add more milk; if it's too thin, add more ice.

½ cup lactose-free milk

½ medium ripe banana, frozen

⅛ medium avocado

1–2 leaves romaine lettuce

¼ teaspoon alcohol-free vanilla extract

⅛ teaspoon alcohol-free peppermint extract

Serves 1	
Per Serving	
Calories	168
Fat	7g
Protein	5g
Sodium	65mg
Fiber	3g
Carbohydrates	23g
Sugar	14g

Place milk in blender, followed by ½ cup ice and remaining ingredients, and blend until smooth. Serve.

Strawberry Morning Smoothie

This filling and delicious smoothie is excellent for breakfast.

½ cup unsweetened coconut milk

½ medium ripe banana, frozen

5 frozen strawberries

¼ cup quick-cooking oats

½ teaspoon alcohol-free vanilla extract

Serves 1	
Per Serving	
Calories	375
Fat	24g
Protein	6g
Sodium	15mg
Fiber	5g
Carbohydrates	35g
Sugar	11g

Place milk in blender, followed by other ingredients, and blend until smooth. Serve.

Pineapple Turmeric Smoothie

This anti-inflammatory smoothie may help suppress symptoms from an IBS attack. Enjoy slowly, and garnish with a pineapple slice for extra fun.

Serves 1

Per Serving

Calories	239
Fat	8g
Protein	6g
Sodium	255mg
Fiber	12g
Carbohydrates	42g
Sugar	23g

1 cup coconut water

½ cup ice

1 cup chopped pineapple

½ teaspoon ground turmeric

½ teaspoon ground cinnamon

¼ teaspoon ground black pepper

1 tablespoon chia seeds

1 tablespoon shredded unsweetened coconut

¼ teaspoon peeled, grated ginger

½ medium lime, peeled, seeds removed

Place coconut water and ice in a blender. Add other ingredients, and blend until smooth. If consistency is too thin, add more ice. Serve.

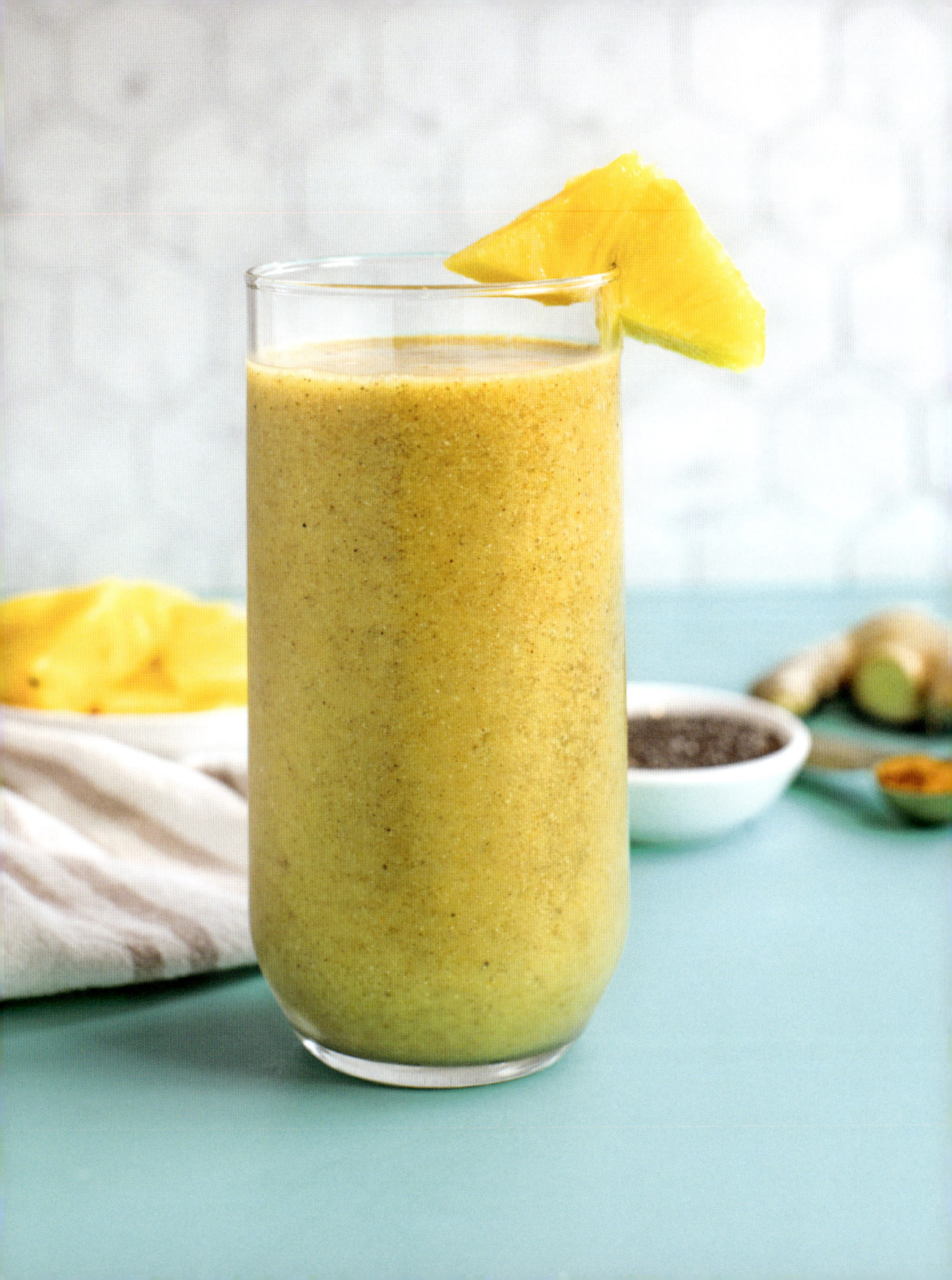

Sample Menu Plans and Snack Suggestions

Plenty of foods on the low-FODMAP diet can be made ahead of time to use throughout the week: soups, salads, sandwiches, snacks, entrées, and more. Though planning and cooking ahead does take some time, it will pay off! Instead of staring into your refrigerator wondering what to make (or turning to high-FODMAP meals out of desperation), you'll be able to easily prepare and enjoy delicious foods that are easy on your body. Here are some sample weekly meals that you can use to help inspire your low-FODMAP eating.

MEAT-EATER 5-DAY PLAN

	Breakfast	Snack	Lunch
Day 1	■ Peanut Butter–Lover Smoothie **Chapter 12**	■ Lactose-free vanilla yogurt ■ 10 blueberries	■ Turkey sandwich on GF bread with Havarti cheese, spinach, mustard, Basic Mayonnaise **Chapter 2**
Day 2	■ Omelet with mozzarella cheese and spinach ■ GF bread ■ ⅛ avocado	■ 1 medium navel orange ■ 10 almonds	■ Beef Soup with Buckwheat **Chapter 9**
Day 3	■ Carrot Cake Overnight Oats with Walnuts **Chapter 3**	■ Dark Chocolate-Covered Pretzels **Chapter 4**	■ Chicken Burger **Chapter 5**
Day 4	■ Turkey sausage ■ brown rice ■ Parmesan cheese	■ 1 slice American cheese ■ rice crackers ■ baby carrots	■ Turkey Quinoa Meatballs with Mozzarella **Chapter 5**
Day 5	■ Quinoa, Egg, Ham, and Cheese Breakfast Muffin **Chapter 3** ■ blueberries	■ 1 slice turkey ■ 1 slice Cheddar cheese ■ 1 cup grapes	■ Ham and Cheddar sandwich on GF bread

MEAT-EATER 5-DAY PLAN

	Snack	Dinner	Notes
Day 1	■ 1 slice Havarti cheese ■ rice crackers	■ Pork Chops with Carrots and Toasted Buckwheat **Chapter 5**	
Day 2	■ 2 small mandarins ■ GF crackers	■ Roast Beef Tenderloin with Parmesan Crust **Chapter 5**	
Day 3	■ ½ cup GF cereal (dry) ■ 2 small kiwifruit	■ Chicken Piccata **Chapter 5**	
Day 4	■ 1 cup grapes	■ Turkey and Kale Pasta **Chapter 5**	
Day 5	■ 1 cup Coconut Cinnamon Popcorn **Chapter 4**	■ Barbecue Pork Macaroni and Cheese **Chapter 5**	

VEGETARIAN 5-DAY PLAN

	Breakfast	Snack	Lunch
Day 1	■ Lactose-free vanilla yogurt ■ Cinnamon Spice Granola **Chapter 3** ■ raspberries	■ Feta Cheese Dip **Chapter 4** ■ green bell pepper ■ rice crackers	■ Collard Green Wraps with Thai Peanut Dressing **Chapter 7**
Day 2	■ Passion Fruit Smoothie Bowl **Chapter 3**	■ Millet bread ■ 1 ounce mozzarella cheese ■ ½ tablespoon Pesto Sauce (made with vegetarian Parmesan cheese) **Chapter 2**	■ Goat Cheese and Potato Tacos with Red Chili Cream Sauce **Chapter 7**
Day 3	■ Autumn Chia Breakfast Bowl **Chapter 3**	■ 1 ounce tortilla chips ■ Pomegranate Salsa **Chapter 10**	■ Vegetable and Rice Noodle Bowl **Chapter 7**
Day 4	■ Eggs Baked in Heirloom Tomatoes (made with vegetarian Parmesan cheese) **Chapter 3**	■ ⅔ cup Savory Baked Tofu **Chapter 7** ■ ¼ cup brown rice	■ Tempeh Tacos **Chapter 7**
Day 5	■ 1 cup quinoa flakes ■ ½ cup almond milk ■ strawberries	■ 1 rice cake ■ 1 tablespoon almond butter	■ Vegetable Nori Roll **Chapter 7**

VEGETARIAN 5-DAY PLAN

	Snack	Dinner	Notes
Day 1	■ Herbes de Provence Almonds **Chapter 4**	■ Mexican-Style Risotto **Chapter 7**	
Day 2	■ Kale Chips **Chapter 4**	■ Carrot, Leek, and Saffron Soup **Chapter 9**	
Day 3	■ Roasted Pumpkin Seeds **Chapter 4**	■ Lentil Chili **Chapter 9**	
Day 4	■ Coconut Cinnamon Popcorn **Chapter 4**	■ Orange Tempeh and Rice Salad **Chapter 7**	
Day 5	■ 1 slice 100% spelt sourdough bread ■ Pesto Sauce (made with vegetarian Parmesan cheese) **Chapter 2**	■ Lentil Pie **Chapter 7**	

VEGAN 5-DAY PLAN

	Breakfast	Snack	Lunch
Day 1	■ Autumn Chia Breakfast Bowl **Chapter 3** ■ almond milk	■ 2 tablespoons Roasted Pumpkin Seeds **Chapter 4**	■ Vegetable Nori Roll **Chapter 7**
Day 2	■ Raspberry Lemon Oatmeal Bar **Chapter 3**	■ 1 piece GF bread ■ ⅛ avocado ■ dash of salt	■ Mixed Grain and Seed Bowl with Vegetables **Chapter 7**
Day 3	■ Cranberry Almond Granola **Chapter 3** ■ hemp milk ■ blueberries	■ 10 Brazil nuts	■ Baked Tofu and Vegetables **Chapter 7**
Day 4	■ Overnight Peanut Butter Pumpkin Spice Oats **Chapter 3**	■ 1 ounce tortilla chips ■ Pomegranate Salsa **Chapter 10**	■ Vegan Cypriot-Style Potato Salad **Chapter 7**
Day 5	■ Flourless Vegan Banana Peanut Butter Pancakes **Chapter 3**	■ Kale Chips **Chapter 4**	■ Summer Vegetable Pasta **Chapter 7**

VEGAN 5-DAY PLAN

	Snack	Dinner	Notes
Day 1	■ Carrots ■ green peppers ■ 1 tablespoon tahini	■ Tempeh Tacos **Chapter 7**	
Day 2	■ 1 tablespoon Roasted Pumpkin Seeds **Chapter 4** ■ 5 Brazil nuts ■ 2 small kiwifruit	■ Macadamia and Quinoa–Stuffed Peppers **Chapter 7**	
Day 3	■ 1 tablespoon no-sugar-added dried cranberries ■ 10 walnut halves	■ Orange Tempeh and Rice Salad **Chapter 7**	
Day 4	■ 1 cup Coconut Cinnamon Popcorn **Chapter 4**	■ Turmeric Rice with Cranberries **Chapter 7** ■ Savory Baked Tofu **Chapter 7**	
Day 5	■ Kale Chips **Chapter 4**	■ Vegan Pad Thai **Chapter 7**	

Basic Snack Serving Sizes and Snack Combo Ideas

Here you'll see examples of appropriate snack sizes on the low-FODMAP diet and also some tasty snack combination ideas to help keep you full and satisfied between meals.

Seeds, Nuts, and Grains

- 2 tablespoons pumpkin seeds
- 10 walnut halves
- 10 Brazil nuts
- 1 cup quinoa flakes
- ¼ cup rice flakes
- 1 slice gluten-free bread, millet bread, or 100% spelt sourdough bread
- 1 tablespoon almond butter on ½ medium banana
- ⅓ cup cubed tofu
- 1 rice cake with 1 tablespoon almond butter
- 1 ounce tortilla chips with Pomegranate Salsa (Chapter 10)

Vegetables

- 1 medium carrot
- ¼ medium stalk celery
- ½ cup sliced cucumber
- ½ cup sliced zucchini
- 1 medium carrot, sliced, with ½ cup sliced green pepper and 1 tablespoon tahini

Fruit

- ½ cup cubed breadfruit

- 10 dried banana chips

- ½ cup cubed cantaloupe

- ½ cup fresh coconut pieces

- 1 tablespoon no-sugar-added dried cranberries

- 1 medium dragon fruit

- 2 segments durian

- 1 cup grapes (any variety)

- 2 small kiwifruit

- 5 longans

- 2 small mandarin oranges

- 1 medium prickly pear

- 1 medium navel orange

- 1 passion fruit

- 1 cup chopped pineapple

- 10 raspberries

- 1 medium star fruit

- 10 strawberries

Cheese and Yogurt Snack Combos

- 1 slice Cheddar cheese with 5 rice crackers

- 1 slice Cheddar cheese with ½ cup mini gluten-free pretzels

- 2 ounces mozzarella cheese on gluten-free crackers (refer to serving size on package) with ½ tablespoon Pesto Sauce (Chapter 2)

- 1 slice melted Havarti cheese on gluten-free bread

- Feta Cheese Dip (Chapter 4) with ½ cup sliced green bell pepper and gluten-free crackers

- 6 ounces lactose-free yogurt with ¼ cup pomegranate seeds

- 6 ounces lactose-free yogurt with 20 blueberries

STANDARD **US/METRIC** MEASUREMENT CONVERSIONS

VOLUME CONVERSIONS

US Volume Measure	Metric Equivalent
⅛ teaspoon	0.5 milliliter
¼ teaspoon	1 milliliter
½ teaspoon	2 milliliters
1 teaspoon	5 milliliters
½ tablespoon	7 milliliters
1 tablespoon (3 teaspoons)	15 milliliters
2 tablespoons (1 fluid ounce)	30 milliliters
¼ cup (4 tablespoons)	60 milliliters
⅓ cup	90 milliliters
½ cup (4 fluid ounces)	125 milliliters
⅔ cup	160 milliliters
¾ cup (6 fluid ounces)	180 milliliters
1 cup (16 tablespoons)	250 milliliters
1 pint (2 cups)	500 milliliters
1 quart (4 cups)	1 liter (about)

WEIGHT CONVERSIONS

US Weight Measure	Metric Equivalent
½ ounce	15 grams
1 ounce	30 grams
2 ounces	60 grams
3 ounces	85 grams
¼ pound (4 ounces)	115 grams
½ pound (8 ounces)	225 grams
¾ pound (12 ounces)	340 grams
1 pound (16 ounces)	454 grams

OVEN TEMPERATURE CONVERSIONS

Degrees Fahrenheit	Degrees Celsius
200 degrees F	95 degrees C
250 degrees F	120 degrees C
275 degrees F	135 degrees C
300 degrees F	150 degrees C
325 degrees F	160 degrees C
350 degrees F	180 degrees C
375 degrees F	190 degrees C
400 degrees F	205 degrees C
425 degrees F	220 degrees C
450 degrees F	230 degrees C

BAKING PAN SIZES

American	Metric
8 × 1½ inch round baking pan	20 × 4 cm cake tin
9 × 1½ inch round baking pan	23 × 3.5 cm cake tin
11 × 7 × 1½ inch baking pan	28 × 18 × 4 cm baking tin
13 × 9 × 2 inch baking pan	30 × 20 × 5 cm baking tin
2 quart rectangular baking dish	30 × 20 × 3 cm baking tin
15 × 10 × 2 inch baking pan	30 × 25 × 2 cm baking tin (Swiss roll tin)
9 inch pie plate	22 × 4 or 23 × 4 cm pie plate
7 or 8 inch springform pan	18 or 20 cm springform or loose bottom cake tin
9 × 5 × 3 inch loaf pan	23 × 13 × 7 cm or 2 lb narrow loaf or pate tin
1½ quart casserole	1.5 liter casserole
2 quart casserole	2 liter casserole

Index